Praise

Medical Cannabis

"Dr. Moskowitz presents an extraordinarily objective and rational approach to understanding the science and physiology of cannabis as well as the social and regulatory issues surrounding its use. It includes a comprehensive description of an endocannaboid system which is in each of us, and how various elements in a phytocannabinoid plant based system can interact with it. This a much needed guide for the medical community and patients with conditions that we don't have good treatments for. It is a must read for anyone with an opinion that medical cannabis does or does not have a role in our society, and anyone who is not sure."

—MICHAEL RIES, MD, Author of *The Joint Kitchen*,
Professor Emeritus, University of California, San Francisco

"This is a book that belongs in every household. It is useful both as a guide to preserving health as well as what to do when illness strikes. Dr. Moskowitz weened me off of two pharmaceutical drugs and their potential side effects with medical marijuana, which did a much better job more safely. We all face physical maladies and pain in life. This work belongs on your bookshelf much the same as the aspirin in your medicine cabinet, which you may no longer need."

—CAROL MORALES

"*Medical Cannabis, A Guide for Patients, Practitioners and Caregivers,* is an exceptional book filled with current knowledge, scientific exploration, and insights procured from working with chronic pain patients and others with unsustainable, often unanswerable, medical conditions.

It explores a path to recovery while openly speaking truth and detailing areas of concern. Dr. Moskowitz speaks from a deep level of knowing from living with chronic pain. He details what other books often gloss over or refuse to address including roadblocks, unanswered questions, collaboration, and other unknowns.

Dr. Moskowitz is a consummate practical researcher, a treatment provider of forgotten patients who have little or no hope, and an "outlier" who always advocates for his patients and those in his sphere of influence."

—PEPPER SBARBARO, RN, MA, MFT

"This is a beautiful expose of the basics of the world of cannabis. It is well organized and presented in a very easy to understand fashion. It is especially relevant for any physician who is interested in using cannabis in their practice. It does cover a wide range of information, including the science explaining how it works in the body and how one would use the medicine without experiencing the psychoactive effects. Because Dr. Moskowitz is an incredible research scientist, he was able to incorporate a large amount of detail, yet manage to engage the reader, people of all backgrounds, especially the cautious patient and caregiver. This is an important work in the newly emerging industry, the use of cannabis medicine. The book even covers the legal basics in various states. Even though the legal aspect is in a stage of development and definition, this book paints a very good picture of a moving target. Use of cannabis as medicine is emerging and still early in its state of evolution. I am sure this book will become an important contribution toward general public acceptance of the once taboo subject. This book makes the use of cannabis a legitimate option, to be used either solely or in combination with other treatments as a complimentary medicine for many different diseases, including use in pain reduction, epilepsy, cancer, stress and a long list of neurological and inflammation based afflictions. The book brings forth the latest definitive information and is a must have addition to any reference library."

—LEONARD LEINOW, Author of *CBD: A Patients Guide to Medicinal Cannabis, Healing without the High,* and owner of Synergy Wellness CBD

"Dr. Michael Moskowitz has written a literary gem that will help patients and practitioners alike navigate the complexities of medical cannabis that hold great promise for millions. The book details in an easy to understand manner most, if not all, of the issues facing patients, caregivers, and physicians in using or recommending medical cannabis. The comprehensive analysis of the endocannabinoid system breaks down the subject so that even the layperson can grasp its importance to our overall health. The chapters describing phytocannabinoids and the use of medical cannabis in different disease states presents this groundbreaking information and the newest research in perfect detail. Physicians will find particularly useful the chapter on dosing where Dr. Moskowitz presents his novel twelve-step plan to introduce patients to cannabis and its uses. His writing dealing with growing cannabis, operating dispensaries, and the legal questions these create are some of the most cogent and thoughtful material that I have read. *Medical Cannabis* is a vital discourse on the subject for patients and medical professionals alike."

—JOSÉ J. HIDALGO, Founder & CEO Knox Medical

"The evidence is in: medical cannabis works to treat a variety of conditions. If you want to figure out how to use it, but want to avoid getting stoned, (or even if you don't care about that), you've come to the right place. *Medical Cannabis* deals in reality, not myth. Dr. Moskowitz steers the reader through the sometimes complex world of medical cannabis treatment, offering well researched, deeply informed, guidance to patients and doctors alike. In the end, you will find that *Medical Cannabis* offers the confidence that comes with clarity."

—SAMUEL G. ALEXANDER, M.DIV., Pain Coach,
paincallsfortransformation.com.

"Dr. Moskowitz superbly defines a much needed, new paradigm for how physicians can collaborate with their patients using medical cannabis. He lays out essential detail about the biochemistry of endocannabinoid systems and then provides excellent guides about how phytocannabinoids contained in cannabis plants can be paired with receptor sites in central and peripheral nervous systems. He provides long-needed detail about potential healing benefits of medical cannabis, which he carefully documents with extensive footnotes. Dr. Moskowitz demystifies beginning, initial treatment efforts; and then guides physicians and their patients how to proceed through intermediate and then advanced care treatment strategies. Dr. Moskowitz's thoroughly-researched Medical Cannabis, written in his engaging writing style makes this the desk top reference for all us."

—S. SCOTT PENGELLY, PHD, Clinical Medical Psychologist,
Eugene, Oregon

"With bewildering claims of benefit, frightening risks of addiction, years of preposterous criminalization and recent legislative legalization in 44 states plus Washington DC, medical marijuana demands an explanation. Fatal overdose is impossible. Cannabis is a safer way to health and well being than caffeine, alcohol, and many prescribed medications including opioids. It should no longer be a target of the war on drugs.

Dr. Michael Moskowitz is a psychiatrist specializing in chronic pain management. He describes years of gratifying experience providing relief of suffering and restoration of physical capacity for patients suffering from cancer, traumatic injury or inflammatory and degenerative joint and brain diseases. His most desperate patients request physical and emotional pain relief wishing to get relief or else to die.

The author represents a rare blend of inquisitive neuroscientist, compassionate physician, wise philosopher and talented writer. This unique manual for Cannabis prescription provides an exhaustive review of the complexities of pharmacological and clinical research, botanical and biochemical identification, physiological responses and commercial availability for various components of medical cannabis. It will be an essential resource for physicians, growers, dispensaries, and politicians".

—PHILIP R. WEINSTEIN MD, Professor Emeritus, University of California San Francisco, Department of Neurological Surgery, Spine Center and Institute for Neurodegenerative Diseases

"Dr. Moskowitz provides a critically necessary reference that unravels the mystery of medical cannabis in clinical practice. He destroys the myths surrounding its use, describes the science and gives providers and patients a resource that will guide the prudent and scientific use of this promising treatment. For the Pain Medicine practitioner, it provides a welcome alternative to multiple medications in the treatment of persistent pain and inflammation."

—MARLA GOLDEN, DO, Pain Medicine Specialist

"At long last, a definitive work on medical cannabis! Dr. Michael Moskowitz infuses his writing with insight, thoughtfulness, and warmth as he parses through the breadth of scholarly research on medical marijuana and shares evidence-based best practices developed in his own medical clinic. His comprehensive compendium demystifies the controversial plant, empowering physicians to treat their patients most effectively and patients to pursue their best lives. As densely packed with information as the cannabis plant is with phytocannabinoids, this brave book stands poised to revolutionize modern medicine."

—MICHELLE WASSERMAN

"This a very timely exceptional guide in HOW to effectively use Medical Cannibis in a personalized evidence-based manner".

—DR EVIAN GORDON, Founder of the largest International Brain Database, Executive Chairman of The Brain Resource Company.

"*Medical Cannabis: A Guide for Patients, Practitioners, and Caregivers* is a quick read, a simplified approach with step by step guidance on therapy, a must read for those involved in patient care. Dr. Moskowitz has taken on a herculean effort to make a complex topic understandable and practical. He has accomplished both these goals."

—BILL MCCARBERG, MD, Past President American Academy of Pain Medicine

"*Medical Cannabis* is not only timely but a thoughtfully crafted and sophisticated sojourn through the history, science and clinical relevance of cannabis. Dr. Moskowitz guides patients; caregivers and clinicians, empowering them with knowledge to better clarify and understand this often misconstrued but very important treatment."

—DAVID J COPENHAVER, MD MPH, Associate Professor, Director of Cancer Pain Management, Anesthesiology and Pain Medicine, University of California at Davis

"Dr. Moskowitz makes a compelling case for both further research and careful medicinal use of cannabis in this exhaustively researched book. As careful scientific inquiry begins to lift the veil of mystery around this ancient and complex substance, we are seeing remarkable possibilities for medical use. This book provides both an up to date understanding of the underlying science of cannabis as well as a practical guidance for practitioners and patients alike."

—ROBERT HINES, MD, Bay Area Pain Medical Associates, Diplomate American Board of Pain Medicine, Diplomate American Board of Psychiatry

This book is dedicated to my wife, Diane Keaney, RN, CNS, whose brilliant brain, unwavering support and hard work transforms everything possible into everything probable. I also want to thank my amazing patients, who have always collaborated with me to come up with optimal treatments for their conditions. Finally, I dedicate this to all of the brave men and women who have worked, at considerable personal risk, to grow, transport, invent and transform treatment options with this incredibly medicinal plant into relief for the long-suffering.

Medical Cannabis:

A Guide for Patients,
Practitioners, and Caregivers

by Michael H. Moskowitz, MD, MPH

© Copyright 2017 Michael H. Moskowitz, MD, MPH

ISBN 978-1-63393-538-9

All rights reserved. No part of this publication may be reproduced, stored in a retrieval system, or transmitted in any form or by any means—electronic, mechanical, photocopy, recording, or any other—except for brief quotations in printed reviews, without the prior written permission of the author.

Published by

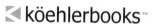 köehlerbooks ™

210 60th Street
Virginia Beach, VA 23451
800-435-4811
www.koehlerbooks.com

Medical Cannabis

A Guide for Patients, Practitioners, and Caregivers

Michael H. Moskowitz, MD, MPH

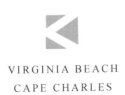

VIRGINIA BEACH
CAPE CHARLES

Table of Contents

Chapter 1

Introduction

THE PURPOSE OF THIS BOOK is to help people with serious illness and their caregivers, providers and their patients and legislators and their constituents to understand the issues involved in making medical cannabis available as treatment for people who have the potential to benefit from it. This is not a simple issue of legalizing medical cannabis. It is woven as deeply into the fabric of our society as health and illness and civil disobedience. Denying it has led to the failed war on drugs, development of an underground economy, a clash of states' rights versus federalism, criminalization of marginalized members of society, racial inequality, and the incarceration of millions of people for recreational and medical use. It provides an alternative to standard care and hope for the hopeless. This is a true grassroots issue that seemed to come out of nowhere, demanding social justice for the seriously ill.

While the current state of the law is fragmented, and unjust, offering availability to some, and the threat of prison to others, it is also a tentative start of a medical revolution. Although there is some excellent and well-researched science on the subject, clinical application is confusing and clinical science lags behind basic research, pharmacological science, and clinical availability. This guide is meant to be interactive and to explain the scope of this treatment, which is varied and quite effective for many. It involves both potential palliation and cure for many conditions. It opens avenues for traditional drug development and plant refinement to solve some of the more stubborn clinical problems that linger to this day. Medical cannabis does not, however, rely on that scientific development. It transcends modern medical treatment, in favor of compassionate use of a plant that anyone can grow and use. Wending through the myriad issues involved in making this treatment work requires information and advice that integrates it into overall medical care. Doctors who certify patients should be aware of the benefits and side effects of various phytocannabinoids present in cannabis. People who choose this treatment need support and advice, from their physicians and other health professionals. Even experienced and successful users can gain new insights that point to new directions in treatment decision making. Informed lawmakers can use increased knowledge to make more reasonable laws that help people get more access to the care they need, while protecting the public's safety. Greater understanding of the issues can lead society to improve its treatment of those in need, including people who have been incarcerated for a substance that others now use to improve their physical and mental health. Mostly, this guide is dedicated to helping those who now suffer to instead live and thrive.

Medical cannabis is not your father's Mary Jane. This is a treatment that is quite different from recreational cannabis. The focus of care is to learn how to use cannabis without feeling high, but this does not mean that the main psychoactive component, THC, should be avoided. It is an important, highly pharmacological part of the Total Cannabinoid Profile (TCP) of the plant and a useful aspect of using medical cannabis. The treatment can never be accurately evaluated with the standard for traditional medical research, but the need for excellent research remains critical. Such research has been in the hands of the people, backed by the states that have challenged the federal authorities. Physicians and researchers must be free to study its effects within strains, between strains, while mixing and matching strains, embodiments and various delivery systems. Its use is supported through all age groups, across political and religious beliefs, and among people with a broad range of medical conditions. Its use for pain, anxiety, and sleep can be superior to current medications, and the whole plant ensemble effect is more therapeutic than individually extracted, pure components. Medical cannabis is helpful in lowering the use of other medications, including opioids, and can substitute for them or work with them, helping optimize medication use to the lowest possible dose. Recent studies have shown cannabis components to not only treat numerous brain degenerative disorders, including Alzheimer's disease, but to also slow down the normal cognitive decline of aging.[1,2]

Cannabis has been used by people for at least the last five millennia. History of its medical use dates to before 1000 BC. This use came to a crashing end in the 1940s, when United States Attorney General Harry Anslinger banned its use with a Catch 22-esque tax law, and threatened to immediately jail any physician who tried to use it in patient care. This was all reinforced decades later, when marijuana was given schedule 1 status, putting it in the same class as heroin, methamphetamine, and crack cocaine. The subsequent war on drugs not only reinforced the nefarious status of marijuana, but resulted in jail and prison time for many people around the world. In the United States, according to statistics from the ACLU, more than half of drug

---

1   Bonnet AE, Marchalant Y. Potential Therapeutical Contributions of the Endocannabinoid System towards Aging and Alzheimer's Disease, *Aging and Disease* 6 no. 5 (2015): 400–405.

2   Bilkei-Gorzo A et al. A chronic low dose of Δ9-tetrahydrocannabinol (THC) restores cognitive function in old mice, *Nature Medicine* (2017). doi:10.1038:/nm.4311.

arrests are for possession of marijuana, and a person of color has a 3.72 more likely chance of being arrested for marijuana possession. Even more surprising, between 2001 and 2010, 88% of the 8.2 million arrests for marijuana crimes were for simple possession. The U.S. Government and many others have spawned an atmosphere of fear mongering, biased "scientific" research, propaganda, and racial inequality. Ultimately this has resulted in one of the most medically useful plants ever known, being deemed without medical value.

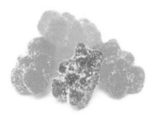

Research has been very limited in the United States. In the 1930s, there was a flurry of research into the chemistry of cannabis in the US, Britain, and Germany, leading to the discovery of cannabidiol (CBD) and cannabinol (CBN) and their isolation from the plant in pure form. This research determined the chemical structure of CBD and developed a few synthetic cannabinoids before it went dark from the 1940s to the 1960s. In the 1960s, Israeli researchers Mechoulam, Shvo, and Gaoni determined several of the properties and components of plant-based cannabis, leading, in the 1980s and 1990s, to the discovery of the innate endocannabinoid system in humans. Their work launched the modern understanding of the medical importance of our built-in cannabinoid system.

Initially, they focused on Delta-9 Tetrahydrocannabinol (THC), the major psychoactive component of cannabis, but they were also able to isolate and synthesize many other cannabinoids from the plant resin[3] (hashish). In the 1960s and 1970s, research in the United States picked up on the pharmacology of the plant, but clinical research remained absent, due to continued legal restraints.

The only legitimate source of medical cannabis in the United States remains the National Institute of Drug Abuse (NIDA) farm maintained at the University of Mississippi. The strains available have been highly limited. The regulations for research have been prohibitively restrictive. The quality of these strains has been dubious at best. The lack of information about other cannabinoids (especially CBD) in both the active and "placebo" forms of the NIDA plants used in clinical research also hamper interpretation of the few studies done with cannabis from the NIDA source.[4] Nascent attempts to grow high-CBD cannabis at the NIDA contracted farm are so far behind the curve of available strains, and the difficulty of clinical research is so high, that it is likely to be a long time before any significant research from this source will be of use. The state of California is stepping into the breach with Assembly Bill 1575, providing registered businesses or research institutions with the ability to procure and store up to half a pound of any strain of cannabis for medical cannabis research. This has been passed onto the California State Senate, where quick approval is expected.

Following California's medical cannabis legalization in 1996, state after state, Puerto Rico, and the District of Columbia have passed medical marijuana laws in defiance of the DEA and Federal law. Currently, 24 states have legalized some form of medical cannabis. Among patients, its use has become so popular that the US Congress attached a rider to the Appropriations Bill on December 16, 2015, stating that state medical cannabis laws took precedence over the

---

3   Mechoulam R. Cannabis: The Israeli Perspective, *Journal of Basic Pharmacology and Physiology* (2015): 1–7.

4   Vergara D et al. Compromised External Validity: Federally Produced *Cannabis* Does Not Reflect Legal Markets, *Nature* (2017): www.nature.com/scientificreports.

federal law. They instructed the DEA and local law enforcement to step down and allow those growers, transporters, distributors, renderers, dispensaries, patients, and doctors to follow state law without fear of arrest or prosecution. A month before this, the state of California revamped its own laws to coax medical cannabis businesses, patients, and physicians out of the shadows, where they could establish legitimate bank and tax accounts, improve access to care, and more appropriately treat patients receiving this treatment. A problem with legitimizing medical cannabis has been a general unwillingness of banks and financial institutions to let cannabis businesses establish accounts, for fear of losing federal licenses due to the illegal nature of the plant.

Additionally, legitimate investment in these businesses ran risks for much the same reason. In California, doctors cannot simply certify patients and then turn them over to the advice of non-professionals, but must take an appropriate clinical role of actively advising, examining, treating, documenting, and following them. The problem is that while many physicians are willing to make a referral for use, they do not know enough about the treatment to advise. This book is designed to change that and provide guidance to physicians based on the most current science.

Another concern is the diverse set of laws in individual states, creating wildly different standards, without any federal standards other than illegality. Furthermore, while Congress has allowed states to determine their own medical cannabis laws, huge legal questions loom about driving safety, interstate travel, underage use, health insurance coverage, business and dispensary regulation, state reciprocity, public intoxication, chemical dependency issues, employee THC screening, interstate commerce, and embodiment or strain issues. This creates a level of confusion with high stakes for all involved.

The ubiquity of recreational cannabis use must also be factored into any decision to use medical cannabis. Recreational use has always pushed the plant toward higher and higher THC levels. Consequently, many of cannabis' medicinal properties have been bred out of these plants, especially cannabidiol (CBD), which tends to decrease the high of THC, without decreasing its blood levels. With increasing demand for medical use, much horticultural science has been brought to bear to change the ratios of the huge number of substances present in cannabis. Doing so has led us to discover specific effects and put them into use. Clinical science, however, lags far behind the cornucopia of horticultural science, and will need to catch up.

Another problem is that recreational cannabis is much more attractive financially than medical cannabis, which may divert capital investment away from medicine. Cannabis farmers are like farmers growing other products: they will grow what is most popular and brings in the greatest income. Some obvious benefits of the huge amount of recreational users' experience informs clinical science. It has led to a great deal of informal research over the years. Side effects and therapeutic effects often merge with each other, and side effects are usually minor and can be slept off. There is no lethal dose of cannabis, which is a great advantage over many of the standard medications we use today. There is also a great acceptance of this treatment from current and former recreational users, but they must understand the differences between cannabis as treatment and cannabis as a recreational drug. For experienced users, a new understanding of "efficacy" that may exclude being intoxicated is essential. There is also a great misconception among non-users that treatment with medical cannabis will force them to be "high" all the time, and that the only method of delivery is via smoking the plant. Even the highest-quality researchers perpetuate this myth, serving the agenda of Big Pharma-produced synthetic drugs that fund their research. NIDA has done no one any service, either, with this propagandizing, continuing to post many of these long-debunked claims on their website and that of the DEA. While the war against drugs may have some legitimate components, the war against patients and general public health does not.

Dispensaries for medical cannabis are quite varied. By far the dominant model is the department store type of dispensary, which stocks products from multiple vendors with diverse delivery systems and colorful names. While the local dispensaries test some products, most testing is up to the vendors, and studies have shown them to be quite inaccurate. This may be because of poor testing, reliance on old testing, the ever-changing nature of harvested cannabis, and/or outright deception. Claims of specific doses in mg may be inaccurate. A larger problem for the buyer at these dispensaries is that the staggering amount of choices can be quite overwhelming, especially to the inexperienced buyer.

Another model of dispensary is the farm to medicine cabinet model. Growers grow their own cannabis and make it into tinctures, oils, and extracts that they sell to their own patient population. While they may carry other vendors' brands, their emphasis is on locally sourced and grown products from trusted growers. This can be a great choice because of the limited size of the dispensaries. The novice buyer may feel more comfortable here. However, these smaller operations may have limited variety of product availability.

The boutique model is that of a relatively small dispensary, using products from other producers, but offering high-quality products in multiple categories with rigorous testing.

Still another model of dispensary is the co-op model, aimed at keeping down costs to the consumer. Co-ops do not usually grow their own cannabis, but tend to work with organic farmers in concert with the preferences of their members. These are often small and are a hybrid of the other three models.

While containing costs is popular among consumers, increasing availability of dispensaries and demand for product already lowers costs. It is important that the dispensaries remain solvent and consumers can choose products they want. Many dispensaries of any type have online or telephone ordering of products available. Many deliver directly to the consumer. These also can be quite overwhelming for the consumer. There are excellent examples of each dispensary model. The salesperson ("budtender") at the dispensary is often asked advice, which may be more appropriate for recreational use than medical use. Budtenders tend to be knowledgeable and very helpful about the plant, but are not medically trained professionals, who treat the patient for related and unrelated medical conditions.

There are literally an unlimited number of products available. How to choose what is best for each condition is an individual choice, but seeking appropriate solutions for specific problems is part of the art of medical cannabis treatment. When is it best to use tinctures, edibles, vaporization, smoke, or oil? What are the problems involved with each method? How does an individual tailor their treatment to give better coverage? When does the social situation favor specific routes of administration over others? How does one develop an appropriately varied way of using medical cannabis? What are the real differences between the colorfully named strains, and what type of variation within the same strain are necessary to understand best use? The paraphernalia used to smoke, vaporize, grind, store, and imbibe medical cannabis is both fascinating and another source of confusion. For physicians, certifying patients for use of medical cannabis is only a first step.

How and when to use the different methods of consumption of cannabis is extremely important. And it can be challenging. One should know not only when it is best to use a tincture, but whether it should it be oil-based or alcohol-based. There are a massive number of herbal and oil-based vaporizers on the market. Understanding how to use these and which ones best suit any individual patient can be a daunting task as well. Edibles can be particularly vexing: their doses are hard to calculate, their side effects are significant, and impairment is frequent. Safely storing the plant is also important to retain its efficacy and keep it out of the reach of children and others.

Cost is an additional issue with medical cannabis. This can be hard for many people to afford. Understanding a specific state's requirements about how much is legal to grow and possess is the difference between following the law and unintentionally breaking it. Techniques to grow and expense associated with these techniques are important to understand.

Some people love to garden and may grow cannabis better than commercial growers. Others may want to try out their hand in hydroponics. What is the difference between growing outdoors or indoors? Furthermore, what to do with the plant after it is grown is an extremely important consideration, as are the various techniques that create safe embodiments and routes of delivery of the treatment.

There are also environmental impacts of growing cannabis for medical use. Commercial growers should consider these carefully. Keeping the green medicine business green is everybody's business and to the advantage of all people.

The reasons for making this work available to the public is to help patients, their caregivers, and their providers to understand the current state of the art and to provide helpful pointers to navigate the difficulties involved in procuring effective treatment. Making wise decisions for medical care is a difficult enough task, whether employing standard or alternative treatment. Medical cannabis treatment is neither. Most cannabis treatment to date has been without medical guidance. It has been extremely creative and, despite lacking medical structure, supervision, or advice, has been very successful for many. This book proposes to "Tame the Wild Beast" and bring a sense of organization guided by the art and science of medicine.

Chapter 2

Endocannabinoids

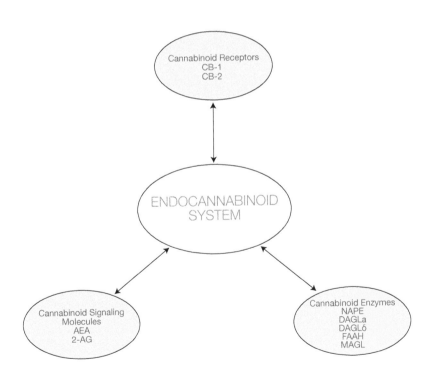

The endocannabinoid system is built into our bodies and, although newly discovered, has been pursued scientifically for many years. It has been far more supported in research than cannabis plants themselves, but even this system has been difficult to research as thoroughly as its important role demands because of the restriction of research on cannabis, the stealth nature of the endocannabinoid system, the need to develop new research tools, and its extreme complexity. Yet it is critical to understand the breadth and complexity of the system that allows medical cannabis to have its effects on the body. This section is written in the more formal style of medical research, because it is important to understand that the statements herein are not just the author's opinion, but based on the best current scientific evidence. It is also aimed at helping physicians and other health providers to underpin their understanding of medical cannabis and how the plant-based phytocannabinoid system interacts with the built-in endocannabinoid system.

When a natural substance influences the body, it is because it either uses or bypasses a system built into the body. The opium poppy works for pain because it uses our built-in endorphin system. Desiccated thyroid replaces and bypasses the body's failing thyroid hormone production system. St. John's-wort works for depression because it enhances the chemistry of the brain's mood-regulating system. Curcumin works on the body's immune system to decrease inflammation. Medical cannabis is effective for a wide variety of conditions because it enhances the body's extensive endocannabinoid system.

Researchers discovered some of the active ingredients in cannabis almost 50 years before they could figure out where and how these substances worked.[5] The first part of the endocannabinoid system to be

5   Gaoni Y, Mechoulam R. Isolation, structure, and partial synthesis of an active constituent of hashish. *Journal of the American Chemical Society* 86, no. 8 (1964): 1646–1647.

discovered was the cannabinoid-1 receptor (CB-1)[6] in the 1980s. Soon after came discovery of the cannabinoid-2 receptor (CB-2).[7] Several years later an Israeli research team, headed by Raphael Mechoulam discovered the neurotransmitter N-arachidonoylethanolamine (AEA).[8] They named it anandamide from the Sanskrit word *ananda* for happiness or bliss and the scientific word amide for the amide chain located at the end of this molecule.

Later, a second endocannabinoid neurotransmitter was discovered, 2-arachidonoyl glycerol (2-AG).[9] Later still, the enzymes responsible for assembly, breakdown, and inactivation of AEA and 2-AG were determined to be part of the endocannabinoid system. AEA and 2-AG turned out to have properties that go well beyond neurotransmission. We still do not understand the full magnitude of this system, but slowly have begun to elucidate it. It is responsible for a broad range of stabilizing and destabilizing activities in the body. A 2013 review by Pacher and Kunos states "modulating Endocannabinoid System activity may have therapeutic potential in almost all diseases affecting humans, including obesity/metabolic syndrome, diabetes and diabetic complication, neurodegenerative, inflammatory, cardiovascular, liver, gastrointestinal, skin diseases, pain, psychiatric disorders, cachexia, cancer, chemotherapy induced

---

6   Devane WA, Dysarz FA 3rd, Johnson MR, Melvin LS, Howlett AC. Determination and characterization of a cannabinoid receptor in rat brain. *Molecular Pharmacology* 34, no. 5 (1988): 605–613.

7   Munro S, Thomas KL, Abu-Shaar M. Molecular characterization of a peripheral receptor for cannabinoids. *Nature* 365, no. 6441 (1993): 61–65.

8   Devane WA, Hanuš L, Breuer A, Pertwee RG, Stevenson LA, Griffin G, et al. Isolation and structure of a brain constituent that binds to the cannabinoid receptor. *Science* 258, no. 5090 (1992): 1946–1949.

9   Mechoulam R, Ben-Shabat S, Hanuš L, Ligumsky M, Kaminski NE, Schatz AR, et al. Identification of an endogenous 2-monoglyceride, present in canine gut, that binds to cannabinoid receptors. *Biochemical Pharmacology* 50, no. 1 (1995): 83–90.

nausea and vomiting, among others."[10]

We now know of a system of immense importance, built into each of us, that is newly discovered but responds to a plant with over 5,000 years of medical use. The current understanding of this system is that there are two cannabinoid receptors (CB-1 and CB-2), two endocannabinoid (eCB) neurotransmitters, and signaling agents (anandamide or AEA and 2-AG), and five enzymes that either synthesize 2-AG (DAGL-α, and DAGL-β), and AEA (NAPE selective phospholipase-D) or break down 2-AG (MAGL) and AEA (FAAH).[11] It also appears two or three other enzymatic and chemical substrates construct AEA.

Regardless of which processes are involved in synthesis of AEA and 2-AG, they are only made in response to an increase of CB-1 or CB-2 receptors in local areas due to injury or disease. This occurs when imbalances develop and results in this system being pinpoint in nature rather than systemic throughout the body. There is also increasing evidence that endocannabinoids modify other systems, which modify the endocannabinoid system in turn. The full impact and importance of the endocannabinoid system is only coming into focus in the last decade, with an explosive focus on research in the last five years. Clinical research remains far behind pharmacological and animal research, mostly due to the politically motivated restrictions that make studying clinical effects of plant cannabinoids like studying plutonium. However, cataloguing and studying the endocannabinoid system is quickly revealing something far more complex than the plant, something that seems to constantly rebalance most of the body's essential systems for controlling pain, mood, inflammation, energy, wellness, and illness.

---

10   Pacher P, Kunos G. Modulating the endocannabinoid system in human health and diseases: successes and failures, *Federation of European Biochemical Society Journal* 280 no. 9 (2013): 1918–1943.

11   Mechoulam R, Hanus LO, Pertwee R, Howlett AC. Early phytocannabinoid history to endocannabinoids and beyond: a cannabinoid timeline, *Nature Neuroscience Review* 15 (2014): 757–764.

A picture is emerging of a system that polices the body's buildup and breakdown functions, trying to balance them. When disease or injury intrude, the same endocannabinoid system intervenes to restore balance. The importance of the endocannabinoid system is still only partially understood, but is becoming clear at a breathtaking pace, with over 8000 articles in PubMed on this system in the best peer-reviewed journals in the world. The complexity of the interplay of this system with other body and brain systems includes interaction of the endocannabinoids with endorphins,[12] hormones,[13] cytokines,[14] growth factors,[15] pleasure molecules,[16] immune cells,[17] connective tissue system,[18] bone metabolism,[19] nerve and glial cell inflammation,[20]

12   Wilson-Poe AR, Morgan MM, Aicher SA, Hegarty DM Distribution of CB1 cannabinoid receptors and their relationship with mu-opioid receptors in the rat periaqueductal gray. *Neuroscience* 213 (2012): 191–200.

13   Lowin T, Straub RH. Cannabinoid based drugs targeting CB-1 and TRPV-1, the sympathetic nervous system, and arthritis. *Arthritis Research and Therapy* 17, no. 1 (2015): 1–13.

14   Bonnett AE, Marchalant, Y, 400–405.

15   Fitzgibbon M, Finn DP, Roche M. High times for painful blues: the endocannabinoid system in pain-depression co-morbidity. *International Journal of Neuropharmacology* 19 no. 3 (2015): 1–20.

16   Mahler SV. Smith KS. Berridge KC. Endocannabinoid hedonic hotspots for sensory pleasure: anandamide in the Nucleus Accumbens, shell enhances liking of a sweet reward. *Neuropharmacology* 32, no. 11 (2007): 2267–2278.

17   Pacher P, Mechoulam R. Is lipid signaling through cannabinoid 2 receptors part of a protective system? *Progress in Lipid Research* 50, no. 2 (2011): 193–211.

18   Kogan NM et al. Cannabidiol, a major non-psychotropic cannabis constituent, enhances fracture healing and stimulates lysyl hydroxylase activity in osteoblasts. *Journal of Mineral and Bone Research* 30, no. 10 (2015): 1905–1913.

19   Pertwee RG et al. International Union of Basic and Clinical Pharmacology, LXXIX: Cannabinoid receptors and their ligands, beyond CB1 and CB2, *Pharmacologic Reviews* 64, no. 4 (2010): 62, 588–631.

20   Currias A et al. Amyloid proteotoxicity initiates an inflammatory response blocked by cannabinoids, *Nature Partner Journals: Aging and Mechanisms of Disease* 2 (2016): 1601–1602; doi 10.1038.

cell regeneration,[21] programmed cell death.[22] We are only in the early stages in understanding the rich complexities at play here. The story has not even significantly filtered into standard medical practice or medical school curricula.

When a system as extensive as the endocannabinoid system succumbs to illnesses such as chronic mood disturbance, persistent pain, osteoporosis or even cancer, figuring out how to rebalance it has great potential. To accomplish this, we need a more complete understanding of that system. The major components of the endocannabinoid system include receptors, stimulators of those receptors and enzymes, in combinations and variations that allow it to fine-tune physical function in exquisite detail.

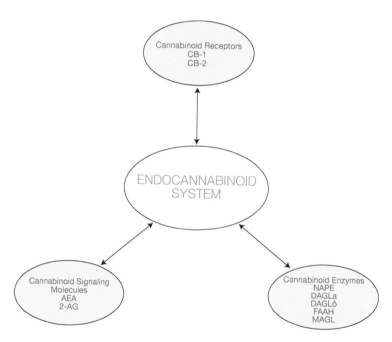

---

21   Shouhami E et al. Endocannabinoids and traumatic brain injury, *British Journal of Pharmacology* 163, no. 7 (2011): 1402–1410.

22   Sancho R et al. Anandamide inhibits Nuclear Factor K-beta activation through a cannabinoid receptor independent pathway, *Molecular Pharmacology* 63, no. 2 (2003): 429–438.

RECEPTORS

The two identified cannabinoid receptors are the CB-1 receptor and the CB-2 receptor. A third receptor the GPR-55 receptor is suspected of being the CB-3 receptor, but there is much confusion and disagreement about this at present, and this work will discuss only the clearly identified receptors in detail. Both receptor types exist in brain and body, and both are activated by the endocannabinoid neurotransmitters, AEA (anandamide), and 2-AG. CB-1 receptors are more prominent than CB-2 receptors in the brain and central nervous system, while CB-2 receptors are more prominent in peripheral tissue.[23]

For a receptor to be activated, it must have a substance that attaches to it and alters chemical and/or electrical activity in the affected cell or tissue. In the brain, this can involve nerve cell transmission or activation of the other cells that make up 90% of brain tissue, called glial cells. In the brain, the CB-1 receptors are quite involved in nerve cell signaling, while CB-2 receptors are involved in local inflammatory and anti-inflammatory responses.

Nerve signaling in the brain involves the structure and function of nerve cells. Nerve cells have several components. Most basically, they involve nerve cell bodies, long nerve cell projections called axons and multiple nerve tentacle-like projections called dendrites.

---

23   Cabral GA, Rogers TJ, Lichtman AH. Turning over a new leaf: Cannabinoid and Endocannabinoid modulation of immune function, *Journal of Neuroimmune Pharmacology* 10, no. 2 (2015): 193–203.

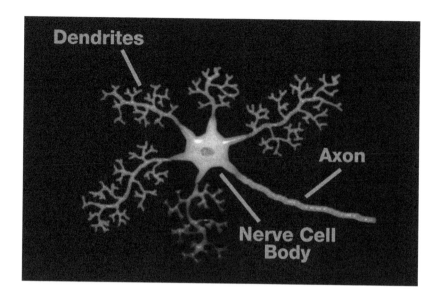

Axons are coated with insulation known as myelin or are left bare. Myelinated nerves conduct electrical signals faster than unmyelinated nerves, which affects the speed at which electrical signals reach their targets. The nerve cells are "connected" to each other at nerve endings, where there are small gaps, too large for electrical signals to pass. It is at these nerve terminals where the incoming electrical signal transforms into a chemical release into the space between nerve cells. The chemical signal then connects with receptors on the nerve endings on the other side of the space, creating a new electrical signal. The entire complex is called a synapse, and the space is called the synaptic cleft. Figure 4 below represents this activity.

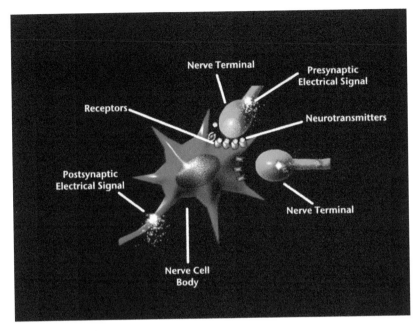

FIGURE 4: SYNAPSE

This system allows nerves to transmit signals at variable speed, frequency, and intensity, creating an infinitely adjustable movement of information throughout the brain. This, in turn, allows the brain to respond to that information in a nuanced, fine-tuned fashion, instructing the body precisely how to change.

Endocannabinoid receptors are located on presynaptic nerve endings. Signaling in a retrograde (backwards) manner, endocannabinoid neurotransmitters are largely nonexistent until constructed in the synapse on demand. As this happens, the brain constantly adjusts to signals coming from the body and from itself, shifting its patterns. The temptation to treat the brain as if it is made up of one hundred billion nerve cells that determine how it functions is compelling, but would be a huge underestimation of brain function. There are nine times more glial cells in the brain than nerve cells. For a long time, these cells were considered to only hold the nerve cells in place, but they do so much more. These functions include nutrition, energy production, network coordination, protection, immunity, and synaptic plasticity. To accomplish these tasks, glial cells must communicate with nerve cells. They achieve this through CB-1 receptors located on both nerve and glial cells.[24] The brain does more than receive information, sending out signals to the body that cause changes in the way we experience life, the way we behave, the way we mature and age, and the way we deal with illness or injury. These brain changes, in response to incoming signals, are a basic aspect of neuroplasticity.

Neuroplasticity is a huge topic in and of itself. It is an important thing to understand, because it determines a great deal about how people function and behave. The brain constantly changes according to input from the body and constantly changes the body in return. As the brain receives signals, it adjusts its own perception and makes changes to the connective tissue system, musculoskeletal system, neuroimmune system, autonomic nervous system, cardiovascular system, metabolic system, and all the organs in the body. These are based on the brain's perception of danger and safety. Unfortunately, in many chronic conditions, the brain's neuroplastic adaptations can be counterproductive and even destructive to the body. There is a constant struggle throughout the lives of individuals between building up systems and breaking them down. Everything living dies, and so the body deteriorates over time. The brain makes micro-adjustments to itself and the body, to delay death as long as possible. In the process, the individual person may suffer from various chronic conditions, all which are attempts to forestall the inevitability of the end of life. These chronic illnesses often miss the mark and hasten death rather than put it off. They almost always add more misery and discomfort.

We have developed treatments from surgery to medication and non-medical approaches to try to alter these processes, and have had

---

24   Chiuchiu V, Leuti A, Maccarrone MJ. Cannabinoid Signaling and Neuroinflammatory Diseases: A Melting pot for the Regulation of Brain Immune Responses, *Journal of Neuroimmune Pharmacology* 10, no. 2 (2015): 268–280.

great success in helping people live with their chronic conditions with less discomfort and greater resilience. We have even been able to put off death in many cases, almost doubling life expectancies.

As we use these powerful approaches, there are often tradeoffs. We can help spinal dysfunction with spine surgery, but the mechanical compensations often lead to further breakdown of the spine. Antibiotics have saved hundreds of millions of lives, but have created problems of their own by changing the bacterial balances in the body that work to augment and direct normal body function. Antipsychotic medications are remarkably effective at toning down psychosis, depression, and anxiety, but cause unpleasant flattening of affect in many people, who cannot tolerate this loss of emotional experience. Statins are remarkably effective in lowering cholesterol, an independent risk factor for cardiac disease, heart attack, stroke, and death, but enhance the development of diabetes, another risk factor for the same things. Opioids are very helpful in suppressing pain, but the side effects of tolerance, dependency, and addiction may be a terrible price to pay for pain relief when these treatments go on for any length of time.

The endocannabinoid system is critical to the micro-adjustments the body makes to right itself when things go awry and to maintain itself when things are normal. The constant struggle in our bodies between breakdown and buildup requires innumerable adjustments throughout a person's life. Fortunately, we have multiple systems built into our being, creating minute changes that add up to prolonged comfort and longevity. The endocannabinoid system doesn't just put off death, but makes the act of living more comfortable, pleasurable, and adaptable.[25] We have been exploiting the body's natural systems for millennia, and our interventions' accuracy has increased with our understanding of how the body uses its systems to control health and longevity. Since the endocannabinoid system is so newly discovered and so little involved in modern medical

25   Mahler SV, Smith KS, Berridge KC, 2267–2278.

interventions or current clinical care, it offers remarkable potential to improve function, longevity, wellbeing, and comfort. This built-in system, dedicated to restoring balance where it has been lost and stimulating pleasure as a guiding principle of all living things, is a major contributor to health and happiness.

CB-1 receptors are located most richly in nerve endings in the brain and body. They are activated by both AEA (anandamide) and 2-AG, the known endocannabinoids. Their location in the brain affects pain, pleasure, mood, memory, cognition, and motor function. CB-1 receptors affect other systems in the brain by changing energy metabolism, decreasing cellular nerve firing, and decreasing brain-based inflammation. They also form with other receptors to modify their activity. CB-1 receptors also exist in immune cells in the brain and body, inhibiting inflammation by slowing down inflammatory molecules and cells.[26]

CB-2 receptors are also located in the brain and peripheral body, mostly in the immune system. Here the substances that act as neurotransmitters in the brain work as immune cell modulators as well. The effect of this is to stop inflammation, to alert the immune system to the presence of cancer cells, and to activate it to attack these cells. Activation of CB-2 receptors tears away the cloaking that makes cancer cells invisible to the immune system, and prevents them from multiplying and spreading. CB-2 receptors are also located on nerve tissue in the brain, but their use there remains unknown at present. When an inflammatory process begins, they are on glial cells in the brain, known as microglia. Anandamide then activates them, starting the resolution of that brain inflammation. CB-2 receptors on bone-forming cells activate bone formation when stimulated.[27]

The CB-1 and CB-2 receptors belong to a family of receptors known as G-Protein Coupled Receptors (GPCRs). This is important,

---

26   Pertwee RG et al. 62, 588–631.

27   Rossi F et al. CB-2 and TRPV-1 receptors oppositely modulate in vitro human osteoblast activity. *Pharmacology Research* 99 (2015): 194–201.

because receptors in this family, including the endocannabinoid receptors, have to be created and replaced every two to three days. This dynamic receptor population allows for increases or decreases in these receptors in response to what is happening in the body. Activated CB-1 receptors influence the activation of AEA and 2-AG, but also other neurotransmitters, including norepinephrine, serotonin, dopamine, orexin, histamine, GABA, and endorphins.[28,29] They are most frequently located on nerve endings in the autonomic nervous system. As a result, they affect many of the automatic functions in brain and body, fine-tuning of everything from breathing and heart rate to connective tissue health and metabolic rate. CB-2 receptors increase during bone resorption and decrease during bone development in direct relationship to the amount of another receptor, the TRPV-1 receptor, which causes breakdown of bone, chronic inflammation, and pain.[30,31] CB-1 and CB-2 receptors have a profound effect on the gut, both in healthy states and in illness. "Virtually all gut functions are controlled by the endocannabinoid system."[32] Stimulating CB-1 receptors in the gut increases gut motility in healthy states, but stimulation of CB-1 and CB-2 decreases excessive abnormal motility in GI illness. CB-2 stimulation restores normal gut motility.[33] Cannabinoid receptors are usually absent in the liver, but when the liver becomes fatty, they are expressed in multiple cell types.

These receptors frequently have opposite effects. For instance, CB-1 activation promotes increased blood lipid levels and liver

28   Lowin T, Straub RH, 1–13.

29   DiMarzo V. Endocannabinoid signaling in the brain: biosynthesis mechanisms in the limelight, *Nature Neuroscience* 14, no. 1 (2011): 9–15.

30   Macarronne M et al. Endocannabinoid signaling at the periphery, 50 years after THC. *Cell: Trends in Pharmacological Science* 26 no. 5 (2015): 277–296.

31   Rossi F et al., 194–201.

32   Pertwee RG et al., 62, 588–631.

33   Duncan M et al. Cannabinoid CB2 receptors in the enteric nervous system modulate gastrointestinal contractility in lipopolysaccharide-treated rats. *American Journal of Physiology: Gastrointestinal and Liver Physiology* 295, no. 1 (2008): G78–G87.

fibrosis, but CB-2 receptors decrease blood lipid levels, fibrosis, and liver inflammation.[34] Typically, such conflict appears to happen in illness-related conditions rather than normal states. Another example of this occurs during cardiac disease. Then, activation of CB-1 receptor may make heart health deteriorate, while activation of CB-2 receptors promotes cardiac health.[35] The CB-2 receptor is highly active in the immune system and lowers inflammation.[36] In muscle tissue, activation of CB-1 may either promote or inhibit energy use, leading to muscle formation or destruction.[37] In obese individuals, the endocannabinoid system gets more active with CB-1 activation, decreasing the effect of insulin in driving sugar out of the bloodstream and into the muscle cells. On the other hand, activated CB-1 receptors are instrumental in bone formation and prevention of osteoporosis.[38] It appears that CB-2 receptors do the opposite.[39] CB-1 and CB-2 receptors and the entire endocannabinoid system play a critical role in male and female fertility, as well as implantation and embryo development.[40] Endocannabinoid receptors are highly involved in skin health and disease, with virtually all skin cells and layers expressing high activity of the endocannabinoid system. CB-1 and CB-2 receptors are also essential to suppressing skin

---

34   Macarronne M et al., Endocannabinoid signaling at the periphery, 50 years after THC, 277–296.

35   Pacher P, Kunos G, 1918–1943.

36   Cencioni MT et al. Anandamide suppresses proliferation and cytokine release from primary human T-lymphocytes mainly via CB2 receptors. *PLoS ONE* 5, no. 1 (2010): e8688. [PubMed: 2009:8669]

37   Iannotti FA et al. The endocannabinoid 2-AG controls skeletal muscle cell differentiation via CB1 receptor-dependent inhibition of Kv7 channels. Proceedings of the National Academy of Science, USA 117 (2014): 2472–2481.

38   Idris AI et al. Cannabinoid receptor type 1 protects against age-related osteoporosis by regulating osteoblast and adipocyte differentiation in marrow stromal cells. *Cell Metabolism* 10, no 2 (2009): 139–147.

39   Ofek O et al. Peripheral cannabinoid receptor, CB2, regulates bone mass. Proceedings of the National Academy of Science USA 103, no. 3 (2006): 696–701.

40   Macarronne M et al., Endocannabinoid signaling at the periphery, 50 years after THC, 277–296.

inflammation and melanoma formation.[41] The endocannabinoid system highly regulates nervous system and brain health. This includes development and specialization of both nerve cells and glial cells.[42] CB-1 and CB-2 receptor activations guide how the brain develops in the growing embryo, with CB-2 dominating early in brain development to help cells establish where they will relocate to form the brain and CB-1 dominating later, to differentiate nerve cells from glial cells and to place these cells in their final location. This also has a major effect on the development of nerve cells that produce GABA, the neurotransmitter that puts the brakes on excessive activity in the brain.[43] CB-1 and CB-2 receptors also are present on the various glial cells that make up 90% of brain cells, and are involved in embryonic placement of nerve cells, structural and nutritional support of nerve cells, the function of the neuroimmune system, development and maintenance of the blood-brain barrier, myelination of nerve axons, regulation of neurotransmitter release, amount and spread, regulation of synaptic growth and development, reading and adjusting circulating molecules in capillaries, activating inflammatory pathways in brain and specific body areas, and

---

41   Karsak M et al. Attenuation of allergic contact dermatitis through the endocannabinoid system. *Science* 316, no. 5830 (2007): 1494–1497.

42   Maccarrone M et al. Programming of neural cells by (endo) cannabinoids: from physiologic rules to emerging therapies, *Nature* Reviews *Neuroscience* 15, no. 12 December 2014: 786–801.

43   Palazuelos J et al. Non-psychoactive CB2 cannabinoid agonists stimulate neural progenitor proliferation. *FASEB Journal* 20, no. 13 (2006): 2405–2407.

coordinating intellectual function of nerve cells.[44,45,46,47,48,49] The endocannabinoid system and particularly the CB-2 receptor are also involved in new nerve cell formation in the adult brain. Hence, the endocannabinoid system is highly involved in regulation of adult neuroplasticity throughout life.[50]

Obviously, receptors do not work alone. But the extent of this system and its specific influence on so many peripheral and central body processes is nothing short of astounding. These two receptors' complexities, subtleties, and influence on so many processes in development, health, and disease emphasize their extreme importance and the need to more fully understand this system.

ENDOCANNABINOID SIGNALING

The two identified endocannabinoids, AEA (anandamide) and 2-AG, activate CB-1 and CB-2 receptors. AEA is less potent but also less discriminating than 2-AG, which shows a greater affinity for CB-2 receptors. AEA and 2-AG are restricted to local effects and manufactured on demand by local proliferation of CB-1 and

---

44   Begbie J, Doherty P, Graham A. Cannabinoid receptor, CB1, expression follows neuronal differentiation in the early chick embryo. *Journal of Anatomy* 205, no. 3 (2004): 213–218.

45   Aguado T et al. The endocannabinoid system promotes astroglial differentiation by acting on neural progenitor cells. *Journal of Neuroscience* 26 (2006): 1551–1561.

46   Periera Jr A, Furlan FA. Astrocyte and human cognition: modeling information integration and modulation of neuronal activity, *Progress in Neurology* 92, no. 3 (2010): 405–420.

47   Abbott NJ, Ronnback L, Hansson E. Astrocyte-endothelial interactions at the blood-brain barrier, *Nature Reviews Neuroscience* 7 (2006): 41–53.

48   Haydon PG, Carmignoto G. Astrocyte control of synaptic transmission and neurovascular coupling, *Physiology Review* 86, no. 3 (2006): 1009–1031.

49   Sild M, Ruthazer ES. Radial glia: progenitor, pathway, and partner. *The Neuroscientist* 17, no. 3 (2011): 288–302.

50   Gao Y et al. Loss of retrograde endocannabinoid signaling and reduced adult neurogenesis in diacylglycerol lipase knock-out mice. *Journal of Neuroscience* 30, no. 6 (2010): 2017–2024.

CB-2 receptors. They are manufactured in synapses of the brain in the synaptic cleft (the space between nerve endings) and are sent to cannabinoid receptors on the presynaptic nerves in a retrograde (backward) transmission compared to usual neurotransmitters. They also can attach to CB-2 receptors on another of the brain's glial cells, called microglia. Normally, microglia are inactive, but patrol the brain. If something crosses into the brain and is not recognized as belonging to the person, microglia activate by growing legs, mounting an inflammatory response, attacking the intruder, and expressing CB-2 receptors. The CB-2 receptors cause local manufacturing of anandamide, which attaches to these receptors and reverses the inflammation in local brain tissue. This tells local astrocytes to stop making inflammation as well and directs nerves in the local inflammatory areas to stop firing. Microglia also express CB-2 receptors when using inflammation to trim away synapses to make room for new synapse formation. To shut off this process, anandamide and 2-AG attach to these CB-2 receptors and stop the inflammatory-based trimming of synapses. AEA also attaches to non-cannabinoid receptors known as TRPV1 and GPR-55 receptors. Modifying these receptors has a significant effect on their involvement in inflammation, pain, and illness. There is also a greater deal of crosstalk, with 2-AG synthesis causing AEA synthesis and AEA synthesis inhibiting 2-AG synthesis.

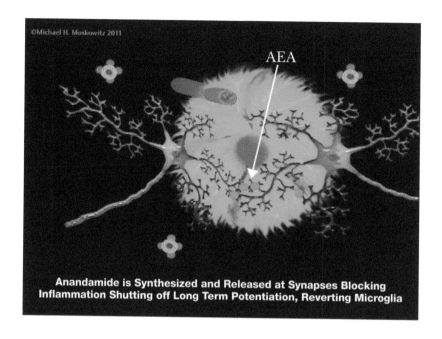

©Michael H. Moskowitz 2011

AEA

Anandamide is Synthesized and Released at Synapses Blocking Inflammation Shutting off Long Term Potentiation, Reverting Microglia

2-AG blocks an animal model of multiple sclerosis, delaying disease onset, limiting disease destructiveness, and promoting longevity.[51] In the opposite vein, it increases breakdown of bone and is up-regulated, while AEA is down-regulated in bone breakdown and osteoporosis. Enhancing and increasing AEA levels down-regulates bone 2-AG and promotes bone formation. It also blocks TRPV1 receptors, which cause breakdown of bone, and blocks inflammation and pain.[52] The combination of AEA, 2-AG, and the CB-1 receptor in the brain protects against neurodegenerative conditions, including Parkinson's disease, multiple sclerosis, Alzheimer's disease, and other dementias.[53] The beta-amyloid protein appears in the brains of people who die with Alzheimer's. Before this protein forms, extracellular accumulations form inside of nerve cells. The formation

51   Lourbopoulus A et al. Administration of 2-arachodonylglycerol ameliorates both acute and chronic autoimmune encephalomyelitis. *Brain Research* 1390 (2011): 126–141.

52   Rossi F et al., 194–201.

53   Bonnet AE and Marchalant Y, 400–405.

of beta-amyloid in nerve cells inflames and kills the cell. When the cell dies, it expels beta-amyloid into the extracellular space of the brain, where it accumulates in plaques as more nerve cells implode. This problem occurs over decades before any dementia is apparent. AEA activating CB-1 receptors inside of nerve cells blocks and prevents it from occurring.[55] Furthermore it has been shown that AEA acts independently of CB-1 or CB-2 receptors at a deep and basic level throughout the body, to block inflammation.[56] AEA also increases sleep by working on the CB-1 receptor in brain sleep centers,[57] decreases anxiety in the areas of the brain where this occurs[58] and inhibits brain cancer. The endocannabinoid system is tumor suppressing in many types of cancer including breast cancer, prostate cancer, ovarian cancer, thyroid cancer, endometrial carcinoma, liver cancer, colon carcinoma, bone cancer, glioma, glioblastoma, non-melanoma skin cancer, melanoma, leukemia, lymphoid tumors and metastatic cancer.[54 59 60 61 62 63 64 65 66].

ENDOCANNABINOID BUILDING BLOCKS AND WRECKING BALLS

Completing the endocannabinoid system are the enzymes that work on the raw material in the body to make AEA and 2-AG and then to break them down. What is so remarkable about these substances is not what they do so much as how they do it. Most neurotransmitters in the CNS are made inside presynaptic nerve cell bodies, and are passed down to nerve endings via transporter proteins. There, they are placed in packets called vesicles, while remaining inactive. These vesicles gather at the nerve endings, and when electrical impulses travel down the nerves to the nerve endings, the vesicles fuse with the nerve endings' membranes, releasing their contents into the synaptic cleft (space). There, the activated neurotransmitters quickly diffuse across to the post-

54   Currias A et al., 1601–1602.

synaptic receptors, and cause the post-synaptic nerves to fire or prevent them from firing. Some of these neurotransmitters are always present in their final form in these vesicles, waiting to be signaled for release and activation.

AEA and 2-AG are nothing like this. These substances do not exist until they are constructed on demand, due to increasing presynaptic amounts of CB-1 or the appearance of CB-2 receptors in the microglial cells of the blood-brain barrier. They are constructed on site by NAPE (AEA), DAGLα, and DAGLδ (2-AG) at post-synaptic areas in the synaptic cleft. AEA and 2-AG diffuse across the synaptic cleft, backwards, to presynaptic nerves, and signal those nerves to fire or not. They also attach to the cell membranes of activated microglia at CB-2 receptors to shut down local inflammatory releases. Within seconds, two other enzymes, FAAH and MAGL, inactivate AEA and 2-AG respectively, returning them to the inactive molecular parts bin, only to be reconstructed if further need arises. Recently, a new part of the endocannabinoid system was discovered. For AEA to present itself to FAAH to be broken down, it is transported off the CB-1 or CB-2 receptors on nerve cell membranes to the inside of the cell by fatty acid binding protein-5 (FABP-5).[55] Essentially, we have an on-demand system that is pinpoint in nature, with targeted receptors, that works on presynaptic nerves, preventing them from firing post-synaptic nerves, and that regulates the immune system, stopping inflammatory releases and lowering inflammation. They disappear as quickly as they are made. These endocannabinoids act like guided missiles, hitting their targets, then disappearing. This is one of the reasons that this system has taken so long to discover, despite its critical importance to survival. This system, while pinpoint

---

55   Elmes MW et al. Fatty Acid-binding Proteins (FABPs) Are Intracellular Carriers for Delta 9-Tetrahydrocannabinol (THC) and Cannabidiol (CBD). *Journal of Biological Chemistry* 190, no. 14 (2015): 8711–8721.

in nature is working all the time all over the body.[56] The problem with developing drugs that block or enhance this system is that blocking it all over the body is likely to cause severe damage and serious consequences to health and wellbeing. A healthy endocannabinoid system is essential to maintain balance in the body, and under- or overstimulation promotes disease and physical breakdown. Drugs don't work by exerting directed effects to one small area and just as quickly disappearing. They stick around for hours to years and tend to suppress the built-in systems they exploit. When this happens in the endocannabinoid system, the effects can be disastrous.

Rimonabant, a CB-1 receptor blocker, was released in fifty countries around the world, as an appetite suppressant and weight loss aid. It had to be pulled from these markets, due to sometime side effects of profound depression and suicidal thought. "As might be predicted, a drug that blocks CB1 neuromodulation at synapses for the major stimulatory (in the case of glutamate) and inhibitory (in the case of GABA) transmitters throughout the brain would be likely to produce multiple 'off-target' effects."[57]

Indeed, inhibitors of the two identified enzymes that break down AEA and 2-AG (FAAH and MAGL) have caused heart and brain inflammation.[58] BIA 10-2474, an experimental drug that decreases FAAH (the enzyme that breaks AEA into spare parts) caused brain damage in 5 out of 6 patients after 5 cumulative doses. One died. Three have ongoing memory problems and gait disturbance. The cumulative effect of this drug caused bleeds in the brain stem and hippocampus.[59] Complicating this picture even further is new

56   Casgio MG and Marini P. Biosynthesis and fate of endocannabinoids, Endocannabinoids: Handbook of Experimental Pharmacology, Pertwee RG, Ed., Springer International Publishing (2015): 39–58.

57   Mechoulam R, Hanus LO, Pertwee R, Howlett AC, 757–764.

58   Macarronne M et al., Endocannabinoid signaling at the periphery, 50 years after THC, 277–296.

59   Kerbrat A et al. Acute neurological disorder from an inhibitor of Fatty Acid Amide Hydrolase. *The New England Journal of Medicine* 375, no. 18 (2016): 1717–1725.

evidence that other enzymes may construct endocannabinoids, that certain cells in certain conditions may store AEA in fully functional form, and that they may be involved in information passed between these cells.[60]

In summary, the endocannabinoid system is a newly discovered but vital system. By maintaining its own balance of receptors, transmitters, and enzymes, it apparently maintains and restores balance in multiple ways throughout the body. This affects widely varied issues regarding health and disease. Indeed, during disease, the system leaps into action to restore normal processes. It is pinpoint in its actions yet active throughout the body. It is present everywhere, yet appears and disappears in a matter of seconds. It affects conditions as varied as multiple forms of cancer, heart disease, osteoporosis, degenerative brain diseases, inflammation, pain, and mood. In healthy states, it helps regulate pleasure, energy, and wellbeing. It has such profound effects that it begs for medications to enhance or block it, but doing so is fraught with danger.

Next, we will look at phytocannabinoids, found in cannabis. The plant offers thousands of years of use with high levels of safety, more efficacy than any of the purified products alone or in combination, and over five hundred cannabinoids, terpenoids, phenols, and flavonoids that balance each other and the endocannabinoid system.

---

60   Macarronne M et al., Endocannabinoid signaling at the periphery, 50 years after THC, 277–296.

Chapter 3

Phytocannabinoids

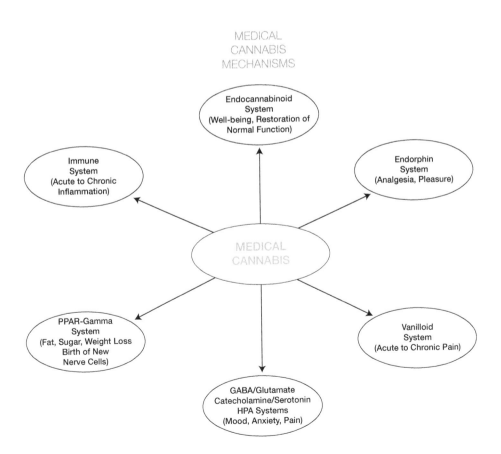

This chapter focuses on the interaction of the biological systems in each of us with the compatible biological system of cannabis plants. As the chapter on endocannabinoids was more formally scientific, with an attempt to keep it accessible and of value for the lay public, the chapter on the plant-based cannabinoids (phytocannabinoids) will also attempt to be as factual as current research allows. This chapter and the endocannabinoid chapter provide the reader with scientific updates of the effects of this plant. While there is controversy about using cannabis to treat actual conditions, there is growing acceptance that the plant has significant medicinal value.

The phytocannabinoids are the substances in plant strains *Cannabis sativa, Cannabis indica,* and hybrids of the two that activate various parts of the endocannabinoid system (the body's built in system). The high compatibility between these two systems is quite remarkable. Cannabidiol (CBD) was incorrectly determined to be a "non-active" part of cannabis eighty years ago, and psychoactive Delta-9-Tetrahydrocannabinol (THC) was figured out thirty years later. While THC tends to be the focus of much recreational use, scientific research, and public interest, its discovery triggered pharmacological investigation that has uncovered over 100 other cannabinoids and many active non-cannabinoid substances, especially plant-based terpenoids, phenols, and flavonoids. Phytocannabinoid variability is complex and matches some of the complexity of the endocannabinoid system. These substances are not the same as those in our endocannabinoid system, but they use endocannabinoid receptors and work outside of the receptor aspect of that system to enhance other endocannabinoid functions. Unlike the endocannabinoid system, the effects of phytocannabinoids are global and systemic, not pinpoint. These cannabinoids have never been found in any other plant, except cannabis species. Ironically, there are aspects of the endocannabinoid system that have been found in raw cacao and black truffles (anandamide). Furthermore, once ingested, phytocannabinoids appear to have a complex and blended activity on the body's endocannabinoid system.

On the other hand, some of the effects of cannabis can be targeted, through thoughtful use of balanced phytocannabinoids toward aspects of the endocannabinoid system. Furthermore, plant cultivators have done far more than develop psychoactive plants with higher-yielding THC levels. They have been growing strains of plants that are not psychoactive or are far less psychoactive, but can be used for medicinal value due to high levels of (CBD) cannabidiol and other pharmacologically active cannabinoids. Preparation of the individual plant for medical use can also greatly influence its disease specificity, especially when developing tinctures, oils, and edibles. While there is no lethal dose of cannabis, phytocannabinoids' side effects need to be understood and managed.

On the other hand, the euphoric high that some consider a side effect may provide therapeutic benefits for others. The idea that high-CBD low-THC plants cover the gamut of needed treatment is incorrect. Although anyone pursuing this treatment must be willing to experience the psychoactive effects of cannabis, careful titration of high-THC preparations, planning of medication delivery route and timing, combining use of different embodiments and routes of administration, customizing individual treatment, and balancing phytocannabinoid profiles can limit or eliminate the cannabis "high." Using proper education and monitoring, a physician can help patients to remain fully functional, safe, and responsible.

No one needs to smoke the plant to get the benefit, but this and its cousin, vaporization, remain excellent, rapid delivery route options. They serve very different purposes in medical treatment than many other ways of ingesting cannabis.

Strains of cannabis have been colorfully named and kept genetically pure. They provide an infinite variability for medical treatment, and the full extent of medical value of any strain needs to be more completely understood and catalogued. Even that is dicey business, because with over 100 cannabinoid components, variation within the same strain on the same harvested plant will change before, during, and after harvest.

One of the more interesting aspects of the endocannabinoid and phytocannabinoid systems is their co-evolution. While people have accidentally and purposefully spread the range and altered the properties of *Cannabis sativa* and *Cannabis indica*, the influence of the plant on our own genetics has not been delineated. The genes we are born with begin changing at the early multiplication of cells immediately after fertilization of the egg with sperm. This *epigenetic change* is due to environmental conditions in the uterus. Our Core DNA is the part of the genome we inherit, and epigenetic change is the way environmental influences, including the substances we consume, alter that genome through our entire lives. Epigenetic change leads to diseases, but also improvements. Cancer is an epigenetic change that occurs from exposure to substances that harm health and longevity. Consuming oily fish creates epigenetic changes that promotes health.

A fascinating aspect of this process is that once epigenetic changes occur they can be inherited by our offspring, becoming part of their core genome. Once people began consuming phytocannabinoids in larger quantities, altering the cannabis genome by transplanting it to non-native environments, breeding plants to possess certain properties, and creating plants to contain specific phytocannabinoid ratios, cannabis began to alter our genetics as well. They also altered the genes of our offspring, whether they used cannabis or not. As a result, our genome has changed our own endocannabinoid system in concert with the phytocannabinoid system.[61]

There are 421 identified chemical compounds in cannabis, over 100 of which are phytocannabinoids. The endocannabinoid system was discovered and named due to the activity of delta-9-tetrahydrocannabinol (THC) on it. Most of the testing of this system

---

61   Willibanks A et al. The evolution of epigenetic: from prokaryotes to humans and its biological consequences. *Genetics and Epigenetics* 8 (2016): 25–36.

has been with refined THC and, more recently, refined CBD.[62] The non-cannabinoids in the plant include many compounds known as terpenoids, phenols, and flavonoids, found throughout a broad range of plant species.[63] While phytocannabinoids are unique to cannabis, the interaction of the phytocannabinoids with these non-cannabinoid substances common throughout the plant world may augment the broad-based effects of cannabis on the body.[64]

Below is a list of a few of the phytocannabinoids and their currently identified pharmacologic activities.[65,66,67,68]

62   Mechoulam R, Hanus LO, Pertwee R, Howlett AC, 757–764.

63   Andre CM, Hausman JF, Guirrierol G. Cannabis Sativa: the plant of a thousand molecules. *Frontiers of Plant Science* (2016): 7–19.

64   Russo EB. Taming THC: potential cannabis synergy and phytocannabinoid-terpenoid entourage effects. *The British Journal of Pharmacology* 163, no. 7 (2011): 1344–1364.

65   Izzo AA et al. Non-psychotropic plant cannabinoids: new therapeutic opportunities from an ancient herb. *Cell Press: Trends in Pharmacologic Science,* in press 2016: 1–13.

66   Brenneisen R. Chemistry and analysis of phytocannabinoids and other cannabis constituents. *Forensic Science and Medicine: Marijuana and the Cannabinoids,* (ElSohly EA, Humana Press, Inc., 2007): 17–59.

67   Rock EM et al. Tetrahydrocannabinolic acid reduces nausea-induced conditioned gaping in rats and vomiting in Suncus murinus. *British Journal of Pharmacology* 70, no. 3 (2013): 641–648.

68   Moldzio R et al. Effects of cannabinoids Δ(9)-tetrahydrocannabinol, Δ(9)-tetrahydrocannabinolic acid, and cannabidiol in MPP+ affected murine mesencephalic cultures/ *Phytomedicine* 19 no. 8–9 (2012): 819–824.

TABLE 1: PHARMACOLOGIC PHYTOCANNABINOIDS

PHYTOCANNABINOID	PHARMACOLOGICAL EFFECTS
Δ9- THC Δ9-Tetrahydrocannabinol	Anti-cancer, anti-proliferative, anti and pro inflammatory, anti-oxidant, analgesic, anxiolytic and anxiogenic, anti-epileptic, anti-emetic (nausea and vomiting), neuroprotective, euphoriant, hedonic, sleep promoting
CBD Cannabidiol	Anti-cancer, anti-proliferative, anti-emetic (nausea and vomiting), anti-inflammatory, antibacterial, anti-diabetic, anti-psoriatic, anti-diarrheal, analgesic, bone stimulant, immunosuppressive, anti-ischemic, antispasmodic, vasorelaxant, neuroprotective, anti-epileptic, antipsychotic, anxiolytic, transforms white fat into brown fat, increases Anandamide activation of CB1 and CB2 receptors
Δ9-THCV Δ9-Tetrahydrocannabivarian	Appetite suppression, bone stimulant, anti-epileptic
CBG Cannabigirol	Anti-proliferative, antibacterial, anti-glaucoma, anti-inflammatory, neuroprotective, anti-cancer, appetite stimulant, smooth muscle anti-spasmodic

PHYTOCANNABINOID	PHARMACOLOGICAL EFFECTS
CBC Cannabichromene	Anti-inflammatory, analgesic, bone stimulant, anti-microbial, anti-proliferative, anti-fungal
CBDA Cannabidiolic Acid	Anti-cancer, anti-proliferative, anti-emetic (nausea and vomiting), anti-inflammatory
Δ9-THCA Δ9-tetrahydrocannabinolic Acid	Anti-spasmodic, anti-proliferative, analgesic, pleasure, mild euphoria, well-being, anti-emetic (nausea and vomiting), anti-inflammatory, neuroprotective
CBDV Cannabidivarin	Bone stimulant
CBN Cannabinol	Analgesic, anti-inflammatory, anti-cancer

Given the above, it is truly startling that political decisions rendered cannabis a Schedule-1 drug, without medicinal value. This is a bit like climate change denial, which may make political sense for some, but totally denies state-of-the-art science. It has made it so much more difficult to understand both the efficacy of treatment approaches using cannabis and delineation of the details of the endocannabinoid system. Fortunately, scientific curiosity has prevailed over politics. Despite draconian restrictions on experimenting with THC and cannabis, the endocannabinoid system has slowly been revealed as one of the most important systems to health and wellbeing across all animal species, from human beings to fruit flies. Many of the remaining cannabinoids have been discovered and classified chemically, but knowledge of their effects is yet to be fully determined. While the United States federal government has decided, as of August of 2017, to keep cannabis and all its components a Schedule 1 drug, it has loosened some of the research restrictions, by allowing universities around the country to use and grow strains other than the National Institute of Drug Abuse cannabis farm at the University of Mississippi. It will remain to be seen how difficult it is to experiment with these substances under protocols handed down by the federal government.

Part of the difficulty of studying the effects of the phytocannabinoids is that they work differently as independent extracts than they do as part of whole plant preparations. Pure THC has psychotropic effects that are partially modified and significantly decreased in the face of high CBD levels.[69] Additionally, in treating the spasticity of multiple sclerosis, the 1:1 ratio of CBD to THC had a better response than either pure THC or pure CBD.[70] In a separate study using an animal model of multiple sclerosis, high THC in a plant extract reversed the actual progression of MS, but CBD in a plant extract did not.[71] In a meticulous study in Israel in 2015, pure CBD was consistently shown to have a very narrow dose range, below or above which it was ineffective, but could relieve pain and inflammation in this narrow "sweet spot." CBD-enriched whole-plant extract, with very low levels of THC, CBC, CBG, CBN, and CBDV, improved as a pain reliever and anti-inflammatory as the dose was increased, and was far more effective than pure CBD.[72]

---

69   Mechoulam R, Hanus LO, Pertwee R, Howlett AC, 757–764.

70   Syed YY, McKeage K, Scott LJ. Delta-9-tetrahydrocannabinol/cannabidiol (Sativex®): a review of its use in patients with moderate to severe spasticity due to multiple sclerosis. *Drugs* 74, no. 5 (2014): 563–78.

71   Moreno-Martet M et al. The disease-modifying effects of a Sativex-like combination of phytocannabinoids in mice with experimental autoimmune encephalomyelitis are preferentially due to Δ9-tetrahydrocannabinol acting through CB1. *Multiple Sclerosis Related Disorders* 6 (2015): 505–511.

72   Gallily R, Yekhtin Z, and Hanuš LO. Overcoming the Bell-Shaped Dose-Response of Cannabidiol by Using Cannabis Extract Enriched in Cannabidiol. *Pharmacology & Pharmacy* 6 (2015): 75-85.

Clearly, the plant extract's ensemble effects, even at extremely low concentrations, was a better treatment for pain and inflammation. The lesson to understand in these and several other studies is that different phytocannabinoids have different effects, but even trace amounts of phytocannabinoids have "ensemble" effects and vary with different diseases or even different aspects of the same disease.

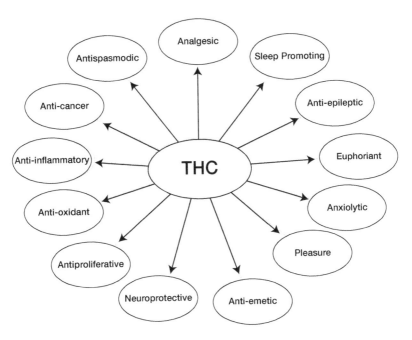

One of the best studied effects of the phytocannabinoids is pain relief. This is where some of the best clinical studies can be found, with relatively good evidence that cannabis is effective for pain control. The problem with the research is that it is not indicative of cannabis as a treatment, only the strain used, the way it was administered, and the conditions treated. THC is the most potent analgesic of all the phytocannabinoids.[73] Its main analgesic effects are due to its activity on CB-1 receptors in the central nervous system (brain and spinal

73   Ramos JA and Bionco FJ. The role of cannabis in prostate cancer: basic science perspective and potential clinical applications. *Indian Journal of Urology* 28, no. 1 (2012): 9–14.

cord) and in peripheral tissue (adrenal gland, adipose (fat) tissue, heart, liver, lung, prostate, uterus, ovary, testis, bone marrow, thymus, tonsils, and presynaptic nerve terminals). THC also decreases signaling from the sensory part of the brain to the emotional part of the brain, dramatically reducing pain by disconnecting its sensation from its emotional impact on the person.[74] This is quite important, because it is the emotional connection to pain, depression, and anxiety that develops, maintains, and connects the chronic aspects of these problems to a person's sense of self. THC also reduces local inflammation in the brain by attaching to inflammation-dependent CB-2 receptors expressed on microglia cell membranes during glial cell inflammatory release. When THC attaches to the CB-2 receptors, it shuts off the inflammatory signals. Additionally, THC appears to enhance a non-endocannabinoid neurotransmitter known as glycine to contribute to analgesia.[75] There is evidence that it blocks several temperature-sensitive receptors, especially TRPV1, a receptor highly involved in acute and chronic pain development, transformation, and maintenance.[76]

THC also eliminates beta-amyloid, blocks beta-amyloid-induced inflammation and prevents cell death, all within the nerve cell, long before the problem can transform into Alzheimer's disease.[77] THC has also shown efficacy in reducing genetic expression of Huntington's disease, another degenerative brain disorder.[78] Two studies have cited decreased intellectual functioning (Meier et al.) and loss of brain volume in specific regions of the brain with daily cannabis use

---

74   Walter C et al. Brain Mapping Based Model of Delta-9-Tetrahydrocannabinol effects on connectivity in the pain matrix. *Neuropsychopharmacology* 41 (2016): 1659–1669.

75   Xiong W et al. Cannabinoid potentiation of glycine receptors contributes to cannabis induced analgesia, *Nature: Chemical Biology* 7, no. 5 (2011): 296–303.

76   De Petrocellis L et al. Effects of cannabinoids and cannabinoid-enriched Cannabis extracts on TRP channels and endocannabinoid metabolic enzymes. *British Journal of Pharmacology* 163, no. 7 (2011): 1479–1494.

77   Currias A et al., 1601–1602.

78   Ibid.

in adolescents and adults (Gilman et al.).[79,80] These studies have been cited in legislation in states restricting medical cannabis use, despite being criticized by several other studies for ignoring socioeconomic status and ongoing alcohol use and abuse. In a newer study done at the University of Colorado in 2015, researchers evaluated age, race, sex, and socioeconomic status of matched adult and adolescent daily cannabis users with non-users. They selected both adult and adolescent daily cannabis users and non-users for alcohol and tobacco use, depression, anxiety, impulsivity, sensation-seeking, and education, comparing sophisticated brain imaging showing brain volumes in areas cited as shrinking in the Gilman study. They found no difference in the structure, volume, or shape of any of the targeted regions or any other regions of the brain.[81]

Cancer research with THC has now extended beyond treatment-based side effects management (nausea, vomiting, chemotherapy pain) to evaluating the potential for destroying cancer cells while sparing normal cells, limiting tumor growth, unmasking cancer to the immune system, and strengthening the immune system.[82]

---

79   Meier MH et al. Persistent cannabis users show neuropsychological decline from childhood to midlife. Proceedings of the National Academy of Sciences USA 109, no. 40 (2012): E2657–E2664.

80   Gilman JM et al. Cannabis use is quantitatively associated with nucleus accumbens and amygdala abnormalities in young adult recreational users. *Journal of Neuroscience* 34, no. 16 (2014): 5529–5538.

81   Weiland BJ et al. Daily marijuana use is not associated with brain morphometric measures in adolescents and adults. *Journal of Neuroscience* 35 no. 4 (2015): 1505–1512.

82   Vara D et al. Anti-tumoral action of cannabinoids on hepatocellular carcinoma: role of AMPK-dependent activation of autophagy. *Cell Death and Differentiation* 18, no. 7 (2011): 1099–1111.

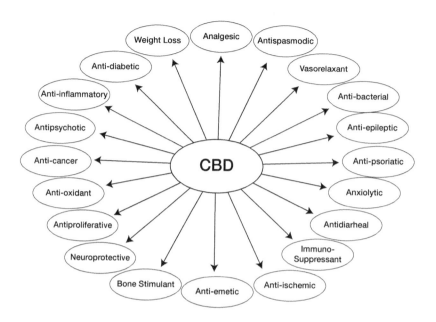

CBD plays a major role by activating and inhibiting non-cannabinoid receptors, as well as enhancing the synthesis and activity of anandamide (AEA) in the central nervous system and the immune system.[83] The effect of this activity is quite extensive, as noted by the therapeutic effects of CBD studied as a pure substance and in combination with whole plant biological extracts. There is evidence that analgesic effects of high-CBD cannabis blocks inflammation processes in the brain and in the body.[84] CBD does not stimulate CB-1 or CB-2 receptors directly and reduces some of the "high" associated with THC, but not all.[85] CBD stimulates bone fusion and calcification of bone, but THC does not.[86] CBD appears to convert

83   DiMarzo V, Piscitelli F. The Endocannabinoid System and its Modulation by Phytocannabinoids. *Neurotherapeutics* 12, no. 4 (2015): 692–698.

84   Ruhaak LR et al. Evaluation of cyclooxygenase inhibiting effects of six major cannabinoids. *Biological Pharmacology Bulletin* 34 no. 5, (2011): 774–778.

85   Mechoulam R, Parker L. Commentary-Toward a better cannabis drug. *British Journal of Pharmacology* 170, no. 7 (2013): 1363–1364.

86   Kogan NM et al., 1905–1913.

white fat cells to brown fat cells, which are considered healthier, non-inflammatory fat, promoting weight loss and cardiovascular health.[87] It also appears that CBD protects the heart from diabetic cardiomyopathy (death of the heart muscle caused by inflammatory effects of diabetes).[88]

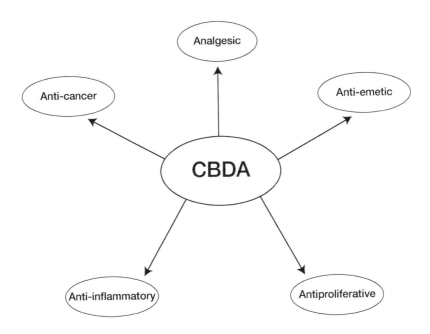

CBDA reduces the spread of cancer with its anti-inflammatory effects and ability to separate the tumor from its blood supply. It also helps with nausea. One of the more interesting facts about CBDA is that the body converts it to CBD more efficiently than heating. This means that the raw plant provides a high source of CBDA, converted to CBD at a rate up to four times higher than the heated plant. This provides dual benefits of CBDA and CBD. Furthermore,

---

87   Parray HJ, Yun JW. Cannabidiol promotes browning in 3T3-L1 adipocytes. *Molecular and Cellular Biochemistry* 416, no. 1–2 (2016): 131–139.

88   Rajesh M et al. Cannabidiol attenuates cardiac dysfunction, oxidative stress, fibrosis, inflammatory, and cell death signaling pathways in diabetic cardiomyopathy. *Journal of the American College of Cardiology* 56, no. 25 (2010): 2115–2125.

CBD breaks down into THC in low quantities, preventing people from feeling some of THC's cognitive or psychoactive effects.[89] Some who are sensitive to THC in the heated preparation are less likely to be sensitive to the raw plant.

THC, CBD, CBN, and CBC each inhibit psoriasis.[90] Both CBD and THC appear to inhibit several types of cancer. A good example is prostate cancer, the most common non-skin cancer among men, second in male cancer deaths only to lung cancer. THC causes cancer cells to implode without activating CB-1 receptors. CBD, CBDA, THCA, CBN, and CBG all prevent prostate cancer cells from rapid growth, inhibiting tumor size and spread.[91] THC, THCA, CBD, CBDA, and CBC strengthen the immune system and are all anti-inflammatory. Testosterone-independent prostate cancer cells, which are harder to treat, more likely to spread cancer, and more likely to be deadly, are sensitive to CBD.[92]

CBD has shown several other benefits as a treatment for numerous degenerative brain disorders, as a solitary substance and as the dominant part of cannabis plant extract. Much of this has been discovered using animal models, but there is increasing evidence that these processes work on human disease, as well.

Conditions include multiple sclerosis, Alzheimer's disease, Parkinson's disease, and Huntington's disease. CBD seems to have multiple targets, including slowing down inactivation of anandamide,

89   Ujvary I, Hanus L. Human metabolites of cannabidiol: A review of their formation, biological activity and relevance in therapy. *Cannabis and Cannabinoid Research* 1, no. 1 (2016): 90–101.

90   Wilkinson JD, Williamson EM. Cannabinoids inhibit human keratinocyte proliferation through a non-CB1/ CB2 mechanism and have a potential therapeutic value in the treatment of psoriasis. *Journal of Dermatological Science* 45, no. 2 (2007): 87–92.

91   Guidon J, Hohmann AG. The endocannabinoid system and cancer: therapeutic implications. *British Journal of Pharmacology* 163, no. 7 (2011): 1447–1463.

92   De Petrocellis L et al. Non-THC cannabinoids inhibit prostate carcinoma growth in vitro and in vivo: pro-apoptotic effects and underlying mechanisms. *British Journal of Pharmacology* 168, no. 1 (2013): 79–102.

blocking receptors outside of the endocannabinoid system that cause these conditions, activating potent antioxidant properties in diseased tissue, enhancing THC effects, limiting THC side effects, and reversing microglial derived brain inflammation.[93]

CBD is low in side effects, and these usually occur at extremely high doses of the pure substance rather than from any plant-based preparation. It can cause a temporary lowering of cortisol, leading to drowsiness.[94] Drowsiness may also occur without lowering cortisol levels.

CBC (cannabichromene) is highly anti-inflammatory in a different pathway then the other cannabinoids. It blocks a pro-inflammatory receptor and it blocks nitric oxide, a major signaling molecule that causes release of the main pain-provoking neurotransmitter, Substance-P.[95] It also reactivates the endocannabinoid system. This is a significant point, because CBC levels of cannabinoid preparations are usually ignored, but they are quite important. CBC also showed antidepressant effects along with CBD and THC in an animal study that also determined that CBG (cannabigerol), and CBN (cannabinol) did not exhibit antidepressant effects.[96]

93   Fernandez-Ruiz J et al. Cannabidiol for neurodegenerative disorders: important new clinical applications for this phytocannabinoid? *British Journal of Clinical Pharmacology* 75, no. 2 (2012): 323–333.

94   Zuardi AW, Guimaraes FS, and Moreira AC. Effect of cannabidiol on plasma prolactin, growth hormone, and cortisol in human volunteers. *Brazilian Journal of Medical and Biological Research* 26, no. 2 (1993): 213–217.

95   Romano B et al. The cannabinoid TRPA1 agonist cannabichromene inhibits nitric oxide production in macrophages and ameliorates murine colitis, *British Journal of Pharmacology* 169, no. 1 (2013): 213–229.

96   El-Alfy A et al. Antidepressant-like effect of Δ9-tetrahydrocannabinol and other cannabinoids isolated from *Cannabis sativa*. *Journal of Pharmacology, Biochemistry and Behavior* 95, no. 4 (2010): 434–442.

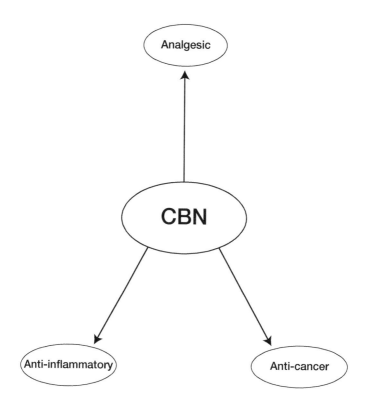

CBN (cannabinol) has analgesic properties. It is found in the plant that has degraded by exposure to sun or oxygen over time in the acid form of CBNA (cannabinolic acid). The body also breaks down THC and THCA to pharmacologically significant amounts of CBN. CBN also has anticarcinogenic effects and is a potent anti-inflammatory.[97]

---

97   De Petrocellis L et al., Effects of cannabinoids and cannabinoid-enriched Cannabis extracts on TRP channels and endocannabinoid metabolic enzymes, 1479–1494.

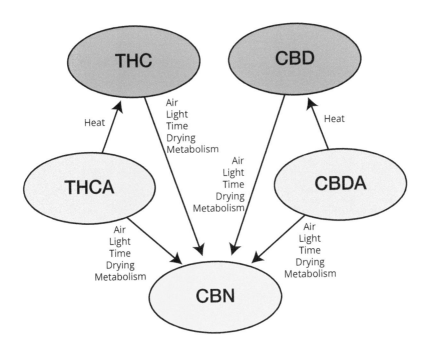

In looking at medical cannabis laws, several states have tried to limit THC content of products sold at medical dispensaries. Some state laws have rendered THC levels negligible, only approving high-CBD, low-THC preparations. The problem with this approach is that THC itself has a great deal of medicinal value, and, for many conditions, a balanced treatment of THC/CBD plus other phytocannabinoids and phytoterpenoids can be helpful. The whole plant preparation has no lethal dose. The speculation is that this is because there are no cannabinoid receptors in the brain stem, where breathing and heart rate are controlled. This is an appealing explanation, but lacks scientific rigor, as there are many drugs, including some of the artificial cannabinoids, which are quite lethal, without affecting these centers in the brain stem. Furthermore, the endocannabinoid system is a balanced system, with each part of the system having effects well beyond mere stimulation of CB-1 and CB-2 receptors. The main endocannabinoid neurotransmitters and immune system signaling agents, AEA and

2-AG, are described as having significant "promiscuity."[98] This means that they have effects beyond the receptors of the endocannabinoid system on other receptors, neurotransmitters, immune cells, and signaling molecules, as well as other organ functions. The same can be said of the phytocannabinoid system.

Therapeutically, this is important as it gives medical cannabis treatment targets outside of the endocannabinoid system. The entire endocannabinoid system (endocannabinoidome) and phytocannabinoid system (phytocannabinoidome) interact and overlap in many aspects, but also work differently than each other in multiple ways. The greatest commonality is the ensemble effect of all the components of each system. This and the phytocannabinoidome's interactions with the endocannabinoidome, being those of simultaneous stimulation and inhibition, appear to make these systems quite compatible.

The problem with THC is exactly the thing that makes it popular for recreational use. Nobody ever smoked cannabis recreationally, to avoid being stoned. The recent developments of plants bred to be high in CBD and low or lower in THC bucks the modern trend of recreational cannabis use to find higher and higher THC content in plants and preparations made from them of tinctures, oils, creams, lotions, and other whole plant products. Ironically, the new plants that are very low in THC and high in CBD are more expensive than the high-THC plants, even at medical dispensaries. Additionally, several studies of medical dispensaries in Washington and California have shown a consistent inaccuracy of labels (only 18% of tested products came reasonably close to labeled claims).[99] While the effects of THC may be pleasant for many, they can compromise work, driving,

---

98   Cascio MG and Marini P. Biosynthesis and fate of endocannabinoids, *Endocannabinoids: Handbook of Experimental Pharmacology*, Pertwee RG, Ed., Springer International Publishing (2015): 39–58.

99   Vandrey R et al. Cannabinoid dose and label accuracy in edible medical cannabis products. *Letter: Journal of the American Medical Association* 313, no. 24 (2015): 2491–2493.

conversation, and sequential memory abilities. More importantly, being able to use this treatment and reduce or eliminate the "high" of THC is essential for consistent and effective treatment. Eliminating the use of THC is not the goal; rather, medical cannabis can be used strategically to block the high when unwanted. Furthermore, the psychotropic effects of THC can be quite useful for sleep and mood,[100] as well as chronic pain.[101] Persistent mood disturbance and pain perception are examples of brain neuroplasticity that has gone in the wrong direction, enhancing depression, anxiety, and pain, rather than suppressing them.[102] THC can reverse these issues and shift neuroplastic processes toward resolution.

CBD has effects on the endocannabinoid system by being directly anti-inflammatory within the immune system, while also increasing local anandamide levels[103] that do affect local CB-1 and CB-2 receptors. This raises a question: what would be the result of delivering CBD with food that contains endocannabinoids?

Two foods containing anandamide are raw chocolate[104] and black truffles.[105] Raw chocolate, also known as raw cacao, contains several substances associated with health and wellbeing. This includes significant levels of anandamide, as well as inhibitory substances that cause anandamide to stay active longer. Roasting raw cacao at almost 500 degrees for 24 hours cooks off 99% of these

100   Roitman P et al. Preliminary open label pilot study of add on oral delta-9-tetrahydrocannabinol in chronic post-traumatic stress disorder. *Clinical Drug Investigation* 34, no. 8 (2014): 587–591.

101   Fitzgibbon M, Finn DP, Roche M, 1–20.

102   Moskowitz MH and Fishman SM. The neurobiological and therapeutic intersections of pain and affective disorders. *Focus 4*, no. 4 (2006): 465–471.

103   Zurier RB and Burstein SH. Cannabinoids, inflammation, and fibrosis. *Federation of the American Societies for Experimental Biology*. www.fasebj.org to IP 169.237.45.31.

104   DiTommaso E, Beltrammo M, Piomelli D. Brain cannabinoids in chocolate. *Nature 382*, no. 6593 (1996): 677–678.

105   Pacioni G et al. Truffles contain endocannabinoid metabolic enzymes and anandamide. *Phytochemistry* 110 (2015): 104–110.

substances; hence, recent studies show negligible levels of them in prepared dark and milk chocolate. This is not an issue in raw cacao.

Black truffles also have significant quantities of anandamide. Unlike raw cacao, which also has high levels of substances preventing the breakdown of anandamide, truffles contain the enzymes that synthesize it.

No work has been done on combining endocannabinoid-containing foods and phytocannabinoids, such as CBD. Would doing so make the effects of anandamide more potent and longer-lasting? Since both the consumption of chocolate and truffles evoke feelings of great pleasure in devotees, and since anandamide is a major pleasure-invoking substance,[106] does the endocannabinoid system influence pleasure-driven overeating?[107]

---

106   Mahler SV, Smith KS, Berridge KC, 2267–2278.

107   Rigamonti AE et al. Anticipatory and consummatory effects of (hedonic) chocolate intake are associated with increased circulating levels of orexigenic peptide gherlin and endocannabinoids in obese adults. *Food & Nutritional Research* 2967, no. 8 (2015): 1–13.

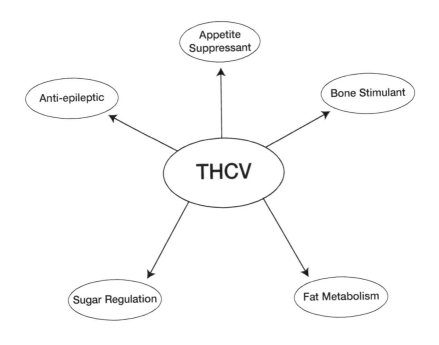

Tetrahydrocannabivarin (THCV) is another cannabinoid found in plants. Recently, breeders have been producing plants higher in this substance. GW Pharmaceuticals is testing a cannabis plant extract made of THCV and CBD in a 1:1 ratio added to standard oral diabetes medication in a human randomized trial to see if this is effective treatment for diabetes. Results are not yet published for this study, but the prospect is exciting. Furthermore, since THCV is a partial antagonist of the CB-1 receptor, would using a strain of cannabis high in THCV result in appetite suppression and/or weight loss, without the unwanted side effects of synthetic cannabinoid blockade causing depression and suicidal thoughts and impulses? Studies of just such a genetically bred plant to treat the syndrome of high blood pressure, high cholesterol, high triglycerides, and diabetes (metabolic syndrome) are being conducted.[108,109] Breeders of these plants have been making it available to other breeders free of charge, to spread its use among those being treated with medical cannabis.[110]

Lung inflammation, coughing, and asthma were all examined with various phytocannabinoids. THC, THC in combination with CBD, and THCV all exhibited different ways they improved airway disease,[111] again illustrating the ensemble effects of medical cannabis treatment. Phytocannabinoids team up to work together to address the multiple causes of lung inflammation. Alone and in combination, hitting multiple targets, phytocannabinoids reduce lung inflammation.

In conclusion, plant-based phytocannabinoids have co-evolved with animal-based endocannabinoids. Humans have cultivated strains of the plant to emphasize different individual phytocannabinoid profiles, and phytocannabinoids have been used by humans as intoxicants and medical treatments for thousands of years.

Each has had significant effects on the other's genome. The total number of phytocannabinoids now exceeds 110 substances. We do not yet know the activity of the vast majority of these. The phytocannabinoids also interact with terpenoids and phenols in the plant to enhance therapeutic effects. The phytocannabinoid and endocannabinoid systems both exhibit the ensemble effect, which

---

108   Hovrath B et al. The endocannabinoid system and plant-derived cannabinoids in diabetes and diabetic complications. *American Journal of Pathology* 180, no. 2 (2012): 180–192.

109   Wargent ET et al. The cannabinoid Delta-9-Tetrahydrocannabivarin (THCV) ameliorates insulin sensitivity in two mouse models of obesity. *Nutrition and Diabetes* 3 (2013): 1–10.

110   O'Shaunnasey's News Service. THCV plants being grown for medical use in California; cannabinoid may counter metabolic-syndrome symptoms. *O'Shaunnasey's: The Journal of Cannabis in Clinical Practice* 1 (2015–2016): 50–51.

111   Makwana R et al. The effects of phytocannabinoids on airway hyper-responsiveness, airway inflammation, and cough. *The Journal of Pharmacology and Experimental Therapeutics* 353, no. 1 (2015): 169–180.

is likely a major reason that they have proven compatible and why phytocannabinoids have no lethal dose in standardized testing.

That does not mean that phytocannabinoids do not have harmful effects. Some are highly subjective, based on whether someone enjoys being high or not. Some are more objective, with too much psychotropic effect causing inflammation and anxiety rather than abating or preventing them. The above-mentioned ensemble effect can soften this treatment, limiting highs and improving the temporary memory problems associated with cannabis. More importantly, the synergy of the various phytocannabinoids, their unique and blended properties, and their activity within and beyond the endocannabinoid system in the body present many interesting treatment opportunities for almost all diseases. The phytocannabinoid system can supplement the endocannabinoid system's job of restoring balance to the body or enhance that same endocannabinoid system to improve its efficacy. Despite governments setting up highly restrictive barriers to legitimate research, the science of understanding how these plant-based products work is now advancing quickly.

While pharmaceutical substances are being worked on and will no doubt be introduced into the pharmacopeia, cannabis is already available in every conceivable form and route of ingestion. Unlike pharmaceutical substances, phytocannabinoids have a safety aspect that is extensive and well-studied. To be sure, there are side effects, unwanted effects, issues of abuse and misuse, and socially disruptive aspects to this treatment, but one only needs to listen to the disclaimers at the end of television ads for FDA-approved drugs to recognize the far greater acceptable risks with these drugs, which are generally much more dangerous than those with medical cannabis. There are disease states such as Alzheimer's disease and other degenerative brain disorders, multiple cancers, autoimmune diseases, psychiatric disorders, and epilepsy, that beg for new treatment. If animal studies with any other safe compound only had one of the multiple benefits of medical cannabis, researchers would be tripping over themselves to make these treatments available. The federal government would have these compounds on the fast track for release for these conditions. Doctors would be knowledgeable about uses and make specific recommendations to their patients. Medical curricula, continuing medical education conferences, medical special interest groups, international health organizations, and insurers would be working to get the information out, develop treatment protocols, and figure out how to fund programs for both individual and public health needs. Instead, the opposite has occurred. While some of this is because the discovery of the endocannabinoid system is new, some is because the medical standard of evidence is not adequate to evaluate treatment with cannabis. It is impossible to draw conclusions about the efficacy of a treatment with as many variables as medical cannabis with a highly controlled, randomized, double-blind, placebo-controlled trial. Still other problems have occurred with selective federal funding for research, skewed toward negative studies. It is long past time to stop denying the medicinal value of cannabis. It is important to find ways to more fully study the traits of all the components of this medicinally valuable plant and how they work with the human body. Moralistic decisions because of the intoxicant effects of some of the phytocannabinoids must yield to a rational approach to explore the full potential of these plants.

The next chapter will address medical use of cannabis. Knowledge of this subject is constantly evolving. These last two chapters on endocannabinoids and phytocannabinoids are detailed and more scientific. The rest of this book will be based on my clinical experience, correlation to scientific understanding, and my opinion. I will illustrate treatment with vignettes of patient experience in my medical practice, and report data from an ongoing clinical case series of medical cannabis patients in my practice. I will describe approaches I have taken with my patients, but am not offering medical advice. Instead I would suggest that you who are reading this book to be treated with medical cannabis, bring these ideas to your physicians. Ask them to recommend this treatment and evaluate treatment success or failure as well as treatment adjustments with you. I strongly believe that this treatment should be done in partnership between physician and patient. I also believe that both need to be well informed. What follows are ideas that should make adjustment to medical cannabis treatment easier, more methodical, and more helpful. While my main clinical experience with medical cannabis treatment is for people suffering with persistent pain, the basic principles are the same for any applicable condition, and, despite claims on packaging or online to the contrary, specific treatment for specific conditions is neither well-studied nor understood. This treatment is so individual that each patient and their practitioners must be willing to try out various approaches to determine best practice. While phytocannabinoid pharmacologic effects are becoming better understood, dosing and disease specificity are not. This is a trial-and-error process that the rest of this book tries to help with more directed trial and less error.

While co-writing and publishing a book, the <u>Neuroplastic Transformation Workbook</u>, and a website, <u>neuroplastix.com</u>, with my partner, Marla Golden, DO, I became aware that many desperate people want direct advice on new and innovative treatment. Given the illegalities of medical cannabis treatment in various parts of the world, I will not be able to provide any direct advice. Instead, I would recommend working with this book and with your physician to help make treatment decisions together, where there are local laws to support this form of treatment. I am also co-developing a mobile application with Randy Perretta that can be used before and during visits to a dispensary. It will help guide buying and treatment decisions, while keeping a record of treatment progress for individual success, failure, and adjustments to help collect enough user-based data to advance the science of medical cannabis treatment.

Chapter 4

Using Medical Cannabis

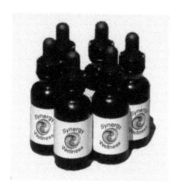

THIS CHAPTER IS THE CENTERPIECE of the book. There is a tremendous need to understand treatment principles and their applications. This chapter is focused on helping physicians to take greater leadership in their roles as clinicians and health advocates for their patients. It is also aimed at the individual pursuing this treatment to try to help them make more informed decisions in their self-experimentation with this approach. People using this treatment need to understand that this is a fluid treatment, because of its constantly shifting composition in any and all forms, in combination with the rapidly changing nature of our own endocannabinoid system.

Additionally, the scientific research involved in understanding the endocannabinoid system, the phytocannabinoid system, and their interactions is continuously unfolding at a rapid pace. Medical cannabis doesn't have to make the user feel "high." Learning how to use this treatment without being mentally altered is essential for those who enjoy that feeling, as much as for those who do not. Plant, tincture, oil, pill, edible, topical, inhaled, swallowed, cooked, raw, rubbed-on or some combination can be used to achieve maximum result, with minimal unwanted effects. Furthermore, using various strains of cannabis can be the difference between success or failure. Since steady supply of any specific strain is variable and that variability prevents the body from adapting to and overcoming therapeutic benefits, learning alternative strains or self-experimentation with several strains can be quite useful.

Another important factor for patients is choosing the right dispensary. This will be covered in its own section, but finding a dispensary that has what the patient needs, while fitting with the patient's personality and lifestyle, may take some effort. Wending through the various strains and their identified effects is often simplified by companies that supply medical cannabis, making specific treatment claims. Unfortunately, these are rarely accurate, due to the completely individual nature of every person's endocannabinoid system determining how they will react. To say that a mixture is analgesic, energizing, or sleep-producing may reflect people claiming these preparations work for them, but this is rather unscientific, speculative, and oversimplified.

THE ROLE OF THE PHYSICIAN

In states with medical cannabis laws, the role of certifying patients for this treatment falls to physicians. The reasoning is that only a patient's physician can clinically determine if the patient qualifies for this care. This is based on the physician's knowledge of the patient's medical conditions, medications, surgeries, substance abuse issues, drug interactions, potential benefits and risks, family history, occupational history, allergies, psychiatric history, and current physical condition.

Unfortunately, many states have tried to limit the conditions being treated by legislating disease appropriateness for this treatment. In some states, it is intractable amyotrophic lateral sclerosis, in others pediatric epilepsy. Since it is doubtful that these conditions are only amenable to medical cannabis treatment in one state and not another, the idea of naming specific diseases to allow this treatment is completely arbitrary and quite different from any other treatment determination. If physicians are given the responsibility of certifying patients, it is physicians who should determine who would benefit from this treatment, not state legislators, the Board of Health, or an administrator for the Department of Health. Given the broad effects and rapidly evolving scientific understanding of the endocannabinoid and phytocannabinoid systems, this is, once again, the injection of politics into science. Limiting physicians like this prevents exploration of new treatment approaches for stubborn conditions that do not yield to any treatment. These can include deadly conditions, such as degenerative brain disease, cancers, and severe epilepsy. A doctor's job is to limit the suffering of their patients, but if the law predetermines which suffering can be addressed and which cannot, your doctor's hands are tied.

Another problem is that at this writing, most physicians know very little about this treatment or the way it affects people, other than holding onto the false belief that most people who do this are trying to escape their condition by getting "stoned." Many physicians feel that this treatment is just a way for people who want to be intoxicated all the time to get a physician to certify them to use medical cannabis. While this may be true for some, it is not the case for most. Most people using this approach are seeking relief. In my own pain practice, we have used medical cannabis to treat persistent neuropathic and inflammatory pain. We have also helped people significantly reduce their other medications, including opioids, anti-inflammatories, anti-spasmodics, anti-epilepsy drugs, anti-anxiety medications, and antidepressants. Additionally, we have used it as an analgesic, an anti-inflammatory, a nerve pain medicine, an anti-anxiety treatment, an antidepressant, a sleep aid, an anti-nausea drug, an appetite stimulant, and a weight loss enhancer. I have advised any patient I have with cancer to use this treatment to try to decrease its spreading and to diminish or reverse tumor growth. I do not recommend doing this in lieu of doctor-recommended cancer therapy, but instead as an adjunct to traditional care. Physicians must learn about this treatment to help guide their patients. To require physicians to certify patients for this treatment, then turn them over to dispensaries and "budtenders" for treatment, is neither clinically nor ethically sound. Physicians need to be knowledgeable and specific in their recommendations. This is a difficult task that should focus on collaboration with one's patient, while working through trial and error toward more self-directed care. Patients need to keep their physicians informed so that they can navigate this highly collaborative treatment approach. In writing this book, I realized that while there was a huge amount of good research on this subject, it was spread throughout the scientific literature, often inaccessible to the practicing clinician. Medical decisions are complex and involve far more than proper strain selection. Physicians should be aware of the different forms medical cannabis treatment takes and differences in time of onset, length of activity, local effects, systemic effects, side effect reduction, and metabolic elimination based on those forms. Unlike traditional medical care, this type of treatment encourages self-exploration of available products by patients rather than strict adherence to physician instructions. While exploring various strategies of treatment is the role of the patient, an ongoing dialogue with one's physician is essential to dynamic treatment strategies and adjustment for side effects and drug interactions. Correlating the actions of the endocannabinoid system with the available strains of medical cannabis and their varied phytocannabinoid profiles is a particularly important role for physicians. It is also our role to keep our patients as safe as possible. We must monitor therapeutic effects, side effects, drug interactions, and risks.

While medical cannabis has no lethal dose, it can be problematic in certain situations. This includes driving under the influence, clinical worsening of symptoms, unexpected side effects, dizziness and falls, public intoxication, interactions with pharmaceuticals, cognitive or emotional impairment, and dependency and abuse.

Perhaps the most important role for physician treatment with medical cannabis is integration of this treatment with other medical care. Medical cannabis treatment is not an alternative to standard medical care. It is a separate treatment best integrated with both traditional medical treatment and alternative medical care.

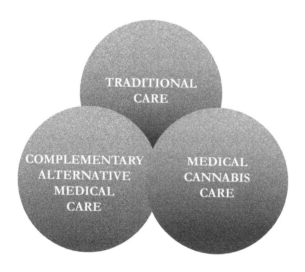

The goal of good medical treatment is to stem disease and preserve life. The accomplished physician must abandon dogma for best practice. Comparing cannabis medicine to traditional medicine is like comparing impressionism to photography. Both are beautiful and can be profound, while neither is confused for the other. One gives the impression of what we observe, while the other observes with precision. They are both composed of color, shapes, perspectives, light, and shadow, but impressionism uses these elements for creative impact that approximates realism, while photography uses realism to express creativity.

Medical cannabis enhances, alters, and exploits what is there, creating something new to restore balance. Traditional medicine suppresses and replaces what is there to restore function.

Unfortunately, the recent trend is to equate evidence-based medicine with only the large and expensive randomized, double-blind, placebo-controlled trials (RCTs), only affordable by pharmaceutical companies, device companies, insurance companies, and the federal government. The history of medicine shows that its major advances come from individual practitioners pushing the boundaries of the status quo to discover such life-changing treatments as anesthesia, new surgical techniques, antibiotics, and epidemic control. These advances all relied on science, but all science, not exclusively the RCT. Evidence-based medicine is about every physician applying science at every level, and using the best evidence available to us to advance the knowledge of the field and predict individual treatment success. Waiting for a vested interest to fund an adequate RCT before trying reasonable new ideas with one's patients is not evidence-based medicine. It is, instead, timid care, relying on "proven" ideas that are almost all disproved within 10 to 20 years.[112] The RCT is incapable of adequately studying medical cannabis, because medical cannabis is too variable a substance in too many ways to be able to draw any general ideas using this type of approach. To adequately study the clinical effects of medical cannabis, we will need big data collection available only through specific applications using huge numbers of people. The government claims that cannabis has no medicinal value because there is not enough clinical evidence to show that it

---

112   Iannidis J. Why Most Published Research Findings Are False. *PLoS Medicine* 2, no. 8 (2005): e124.

does have value. This is only based on a dearth of RCTs, because the clinical evidence is overwhelmingly clear that cannabis is likely to have more clinical value than any plant in history, including willow bark (aspirin), foxglove (warfarin), and the poppy (opium).

Medical cannabis treatment has presented physicians with an opportunity to participate in their patients' care with a medicinally valuable, non-lethal substance and to integrate that treatment with the rest of their care. It will be many years before understanding of the endocannabinoid system will find its way into medical school teaching and step into the limelight as a therapeutic target. Hopefully, by then, enough physicians will have become experienced in this treatment to lead the way for the rest.

THE ROLE OF THE PATIENT

In most states, once a patient is certified, they are on their own. After a patient finds and is certified by a physician, they must locate and join a dispensary; figure out what type of cannabis they wish to try; determine how to integrate it with their traditional and complementary medical care; try several different strains, embodiments, and schedules of use; find out about the drug testing policies of their workplace and whether a doctor's certification protects them from disciplinary action; find out about how to mix and match different aspects of treatment; establish which types of medical cannabis treatment works best for their condition; and learn how to use this without psychological alteration or cognitive impairment. That is quite a lot to expect from a patient. Making the budtender (salesperson) at a dispensary a de facto cannabis practitioner is not appropriate. Budtenders are often very knowledgeable about strains, but most of that knowledge is THC-oriented. Patients already believe incorrectly that if they are not altered, the cannabis is ineffective. Despite all this, vast numbers of people have figured out how to do this treatment with excellent results through trial and error, based on limited advice from dispensaries, books, the internet, friends, and family members. This is a positive aspect to this approach, because it is highly adaptable, forgiving, and interactive and helps individuals determine what works best for them. More directed selection of choice with the guidance of one's practitioner can make a huge difference in both the start and success of this treatment. It is important to have people try things beyond those recommended by the treating doctor. Patients must be willing to risk being intoxicated to find their limits and to determine if they can cancel this effect if it is unwanted. Any intoxication is usually limited to a few hours and/or resolves with sleep.

The way physicians gain understanding of the effects of any treatment, which is critical to success, is via patient feedback. Studies tend to test products under idealized conditions, but the real value of any treatment is determined in the much more complex real world in which we all live. People take multiple medications and supplements. They have variable individual responses to treatment. They come with different genetic backgrounds and preconceived ideas. They often have many medical problems that may respond positively or negatively to any one treatment. Different people may follow physician recommendations and instructions in different ways. Lack or success of response tends to determine on-the-spot dose adjustments. Social stress can significantly interfere with most treatments. Financial considerations must be considered, as must self-monitoring for responsible use. Any patient's tendency toward active or passive participation in medical care is yet another variable. Family attitudes toward treatment can have a profound effect on outcome. Substance abuse issues often need to be considered. Firing up a joint or a pipe is far less socially acceptable than taking a capsule. Understanding these and other factors in a treatment with a substance as variable as medical cannabis can be difficult to figure out.

One role that patients can help with is data collection. Paying attention to response for symptoms, side effects, mood changes, anxiety responses, and quality of life issues can help determine the value of this treatment approach for any individual. This will also help the patient's collaborating physician to understand outcome and to make positive recommendations. In my pain practice, I keep a database of responses for patients treated with medical cannabis. These include whether the following is unchanged, improved or worse:

Pain

Sleep

Stress

Quality of Life

Energy

Focus

Opioid reduction for patients taking these medications

Substituting or adding any other symptom for pain is reasonable, depending on what is being treated. We also look for side effects and catalogue these, as well. Looking at this can help determine responsiveness of treatment, as well as when and which adjustments to make. As stated before, treatment with cannabis is infinitely adjustable. This can be a passive process for the user, relying on the internally changing nature of both phytocannabinoids and endocannabinoids. It can also be purposefully directed, allowing for more precise treatment decisions and effective changes. Key to understanding is to pick a set of symptoms and to gather information about personal response. We need to develop apps that can let users collect this information and upload it to a central source to be evaluated. This can also be invaluable to improving the specificity of treatment recommendations. Appropriate safeguards of participant anonymity and confidentiality are a critical aspect of this type of application.

Note that the above list of problems is a general one, not disease-specific. This is an important issue with medical cannabis as a treatment. This is a treatment approach aimed at restoring normal balance in multiple systems throughout the body. While it has potential applicability to a broad spectrum of diseases, the goal of this treatment is restoration of health and wellbeing through symptom reduction. It utilizes the endocannabinoid system's ability to mediate itself and multiple other systems to re-establish pain control, mood stability, healthy metabolic rate, new nerve cell growth and development, normalized immune system response, wellbeing, and pleasure.

The patient can also exploit the variability of medical cannabis and its interaction with our own endocannabinoid system. Openness to trying new approaches can be quite helpful. The advantage of a constantly shifting internal and external mix of endocannabinoids and phytocannabinoids is that the body does not become tolerant to any one approach, making it harder for disease to express itself in the face of this constantly adjusting treatment. Because the phytocannabinoids strengthen and enhance the endocannabinoid system, then work on the same system they have activated and improved, the chance to create profound internal changes in chronic illness is significant. In chronic conditions, the body resets to survive within the relentlessness of the disease. With a treatment that constantly shifts its own milieu and the body's internal milieu, combined with such broad-based anti-inflammatory and neuroprotective traits, we have a real chance of making fundamental changes. For the patient, establishing effective care, then trying new and varied products can be extremely helpful.

RECREATIONAL VERSUS MEDICAL

The purpose of recreational cannabis is to experience an altered state known by many names: getting stoned, getting high, being zonked, etc. The purpose of medical cannabis is to get well. Being stoned is a possibility, but the focus is on how to use this as effective treatment without being altered. This difference goes deep into this treatment, from plant genetics to developing various approaches to using all forms of the plant with the express purpose of not getting high. But why would anyone use a plant that is famous for its high with the express purpose of not being stoned? Because medical treatment that alters consciousness is neither desirable nor sustainable.

TABLE 2: RECREATIONAL VS MEDICAL CANNABIS

	RECREATIONAL	MEDICAL
Purpose	Being altered	Getting Well
Strains	High THC, low CBD, other phytocannabinoids are ignored	HIGH CBD, CBDA, THCA, THC, CBG, CBC, CBN, CBDV, THCV
Temperature	Always heated or preheated	Heated, preheated, raw and fresh

	RECREATIONAL	MEDICAL
Desirable Effects	Well-being, euphoria, sensory enhancement, relaxation, pleasure, soothing, fun, laughter, mild hallucinations	Symptom relief, nudging body back to normal, reduction of illness burden, well-being, improved pain control, improved sleep, improved energy, improved focus, improved quality of life, improved stress management, reduction of medications, pleasure, soothing, protection of the nervous system, improved immune function, appetite regulation
Undesirable Side Effects	Not being altered, dizziness, anxiety, panic, loss of motivation, dry mouth, confusion, risk of arrest, fines and imprisonment	Being altered when not appropriate, interference with social activities, dizziness, anxiety, panic, loss of motivation, dry mouth, confusion, risk of arrest, fines and imprisonment

These distinctions are particularly important, because the realities of each are often contrary to the other. Recreational cannabis has been "legalized" in several states, but this status is quite tenuous, depending on who is enforcing federal and state law. Treatment and law enforcement often come into conflict with each other. Lawmakers often lack understanding of the potential benefits of cannabis treatment, approving varied laws or keeping medical use illegal. Even states that have strong medical use must contend with federal laws that make it impossible for the treatment's business aspects to flourish. Medical issues addressed by cannabis are just as valid in states that do not have medical cannabis laws as in states that do. These laws vary so much between states that treatment must be hewed together based on legislative variations, rather than disease and burden of illness considerations. On the other hand, many who use medical cannabis are just doing so for recreation, casting a shadow over medical users as just wanting to get high. Helping inexperienced users figure out how to use this treatment to get desirable medical benefits and avoid undesirable side effects requires debunking the myth of being high, not to mention a daunting education in acquisition, preparation, and appropriate use. The difficulty with experienced users is in helping them understand that if a treatment does not get the user high, it can still be effective treatment.

Recreational use is much more profitable than current medical use and involves a great deal more of state populations. Everything from tax revenues for states to prices that growers can get for high-THC plants versus low-THC plants makes medical cannabis treatment either a legal way to get around illegal recreational use or the stepchild of recreational use. Physicians do not want to be associated with recreational cannabis, so they avoid medical use with their patients. As a result, this complex and nuanced treatment is given far less shrift than complementary and alternative medical treatments that lack any scientific rigor compared to the robust science behind medical cannabis use. The gift of medical care is physician-led guidance to manage and relieve illness, while discovering, exploring, organizing, and managing treatment. Medical cannabis treatment has largely been left to experienced users, whose main exposure to it has been recreational. As a result, disease and treatment advice are often lacking and are skewed toward getting high.

Conditions That May Respond to Medical Cannabis Treatment

This section starts with a caution. There is excellent scientific evidence that medical cannabis can help many types of medical illness, but scant medical evidence. The lack of medical evidence does not signify a lack of efficacy. While there tend to be a few small RCTs, the "gold standard" of medical evidence, there are multiple other forms of evidence that are just as, if not more compelling, under variable circumstances. Looking at medical evidence, we must consider a broad array of collecting and evaluating data. The basic research that goes into discovering the science that predicts clinical use is a critical starting point for gathering evidence. The case studies of people showing improvement with treatment is another important data set. The retrospective review of individuals who have responded to treatment and large population studies of different ways of treating the condition being studied represent two more ways to examine the evidence. Medical chart review of practitioners' ongoing patients receiving the treatment allows multiple medical practices to compare treatment results. Exploring pharmacological studies of the individual components of the treatment to determine their specific, additive, and synergistic mechanisms of action leads to critical aspects of clinical evidence. Safety of the treatment and review of unexpected or newly emerging treatment outcomes are most important to ensuring lasting treatment success. The use of large data collection through mobile applications and use of computerized neural networks to evaluate multiple variables of long-term treatment allows for far greater "real world" evidence than the usual 8- to 16-week Randomized Controlled Trial. The point is that when all this evidence is looked at for medical cannabis, the endocannabinoid system, and the phytocannabinoid system, what emerges is a treatment based on best available evidence that is effective, safe, and in need of more study.

There is evidence that medical cannabis is an effective treatment for multiple medical disorders and symptoms. The best current evidence shows that medical cannabis can be useful for treating acute and chronic pain, anxiety, nausea, vomiting, appetite loss, obesity, chemotherapy induced side effects, brain injury, brain inflammation, cancer, diabetic heart damage, major depression, liver toxicity, arthritis, auto-immune disorders, post-traumatic stress disorder, degenerative brain disorders, inflammatory bowel disease, metabolic syndrome, epilepsy, insomnia, skin disorders, osteoporosis, neuropathy, psychosis, infections, muscle spasm, and inflammation. Even if further study shows that most of these conditions are not helped by treatment with medical cannabis, the remaining list of conditions helped would be astonishing. The issue remaining is not whether a specific strain of medical cannabis fails to relieve any of these conditions, but which strains, combinations of strains, different routes of administration, varied embodiments of medical cannabis, and combinations of medical cannabis treatment, traditional treatment, and complementary and alternative treatment work best to relieve and cure these conditions. This complexity of care is another compelling reason for physicians to become increasingly involved with their patients in selection, adjustment, and direction of care.

There is another reported phenomenon of medical cannabis treatment: the reduction of pain medications by people receiving it. The value of reducing the use of pain medications for pain patients is huge. This is not limited to opioid medications. It involves medications from all classes, including opioids, nerve pain medicines, antidepressants, anti-inflammatories, sleeping medications, anti-anxiety drugs, and anti-spasmodics. A study of Part D Medicare prescription use in states that have medical cannabis laws from 2010 to 2013 showed a 25% decrease in the sale of pharmaceuticals for which cannabis could substitute. This same study showed a 2013-estimated $165.2 million in savings from use of medical cannabis in Medicare Part D drug payments to those states with medical cannabis laws.[113] Basically, people are paying out of pocket for their own care while eliminating high amounts of pharmaceutical costs and consumption. Medical cannabis, this federally repudiated, largely unsupervised, and personally expensive treatment, has resulted in self-procured care in a patient-directed system. While medical cannabis is used with traditional care, its ragtag, sputtering use has many people pulling back on pharmaceuticals and outflanking the insurance industry. Imagine if this treatment had the backing of the federal government in all fifty states, with well-informed physicians guiding their self-empowered patients. Anyone can grow this plant for relatively little cost to supply their own needs. The savings would be incredible.

Collaborative work with physicians and patients would improve. Consumer choice for which and how much of each type of care to choose would expand, with competition spawning more consumer savings.

THE UNSTONED

The misconception that medical cannabis is all about getting "high" due to the psychotropic effects of THC must be reconsidered. There are forms of the plant and ways to take it that do not introduce significant amounts of THC into the system, deliver alternative phytocannabinoids, block THC effects, and/or use the body's own metabolic systems to prevent THC transformation from THCA. Each strategy incorporates the ensemble effects of the phytocannabinoids and should be first tried in the 3–5-hour period before sleep, in order to avoid being at work or behind the wheel of a car before gauging effects and side effects. Some delivery methods of consuming cannabis can manifest their effects in minutes, but most

---

113   Bradford AC, Bradford WD. Medical Marijuana Laws Reduce Prescription Medication Use In Medicare Part D. *Health Affairs* 35, no. 7 (2016): 1230–1236.

orally ingested forms will take 1–2 hours to take effect. Starting with a high-CBD, low-THC strain is best, whether a person is experienced using cannabis for recreational purposes or not. Most of the cannabis used for recreational purposes is very low in CBD, because CBD can cancel out much of the "high" associated with THC ingestion. I would recommend finding an 18:1 to 26:1 CBD:THC strain of cannabis. These can be hard to locate as flowers or buds, but are easier to find as tinctures and as concentrated vaporization oil. The reason to start with this is that the vast majority of people do not want to get "high" on this medication or prefer to determine how, when, and where they will experience those consciousness-altering effects. Although the THC in medical cannabis provides many of the benefit of that molecule, high CBD-to-THC ratios result in CBD canceling out many of the psychotropic effects of THC, without lowering its body or tissue levels.

One caution is about product testing. Much testing is done with batches that were grown or processed long before the current available batch, and label accuracy is often difficult to determine. Knowing how recently testing was performed can help. Reading the label is critical, because advice is often inaccurate and the label at least points in the right direction.

TABLE 3: METHODS OF USING MEDICAL CANNABIS WITHOUT COGNITIVE IMPAIRMENT

APPROACH	CANNABIS EMBODIMENT
Heated	High CBD and Low THC smoked, vaped, capsules, concentrated oil, tinctures, preheated in the oven
Raw	Any strain can be used in capsule, smoothie, salad. Always test at non-critical time
Titration	Tincture (High CBD Low THC), capsule, salad, smoothie or in other uncooked food (any strain)
During Sleep	THC. CBD, tinctures, raw capsule, smoothie, salad, concentrated oil, vaporize to initiate sleep, oral consumption to maintain sleep
Morning Hangover	Vaporize high CBD low THC
Topical	Lotions, creams, salves, shampoos, conditioner, soaps
In Mouth	Tincture of high CBD, high THC or combination of both rubbed on muscle in the cheek

The psychotropic effects of cannabis are due to THC. Many people enjoy these effects, and they can be medically beneficial, but for others, they can be problematic. This book is not aimed at avoiding THC effects at all costs. In fact, the potential benefits of THC are nothing short of remarkable. The issue is that these psychotropic effects are not appropriate in many important situations in people's lives, and if using medical cannabis involved being "high" all the time, the treatment would have far less usefulness. It is critical that anyone wishing to try medical cannabis learn how not to be "high," so that the part of life requiring unaltered states of consciousness can be seamlessly experienced and thoroughly enjoyed. Medical cannabis treatment is most effective with a balanced intake of the various phytocannabinoids, terpenoids, phenols, and flavonoids in the cannabis plant. Focusing on only one component or strain of the plant is limiting and gives too much chance for the treated illness or injury to adapt and overcome effectiveness. The body's ability to do this is the unfortunate fact of most treatment. One advantage of using variable treatment is that the body has a difficult time adapting around a constantly variable set of phytocannabinoids and their ratios to each other.

Chronic medical disease is a compromise that often prolongs life and puts off death. Brain and body will strive to maintain the condition, because the alternative involves the real or potential threat of death, and both fight this off at all costs. When the condition overwhelms the body's healing and palliative processes, a great deal of effort is spent keeping the body going, even at the cost of one's comfort and wellbeing. A varied palette of phytocannabinoids gives the treatment a chance to stay ahead of the body's ability to adapt and maintain disease states. Fortunately, the plant's own constantly shifting ratios of substances is helpful, but bigger variations developed by individual patients are likely to be even more effective. This is not like treatment with pharmaceuticals. Medications are stable compounds, often unchanged in potency for decades after expiration dates. Cannabis starts to change as soon as it is harvested and keeps changing until it is fully consumed. This changing profile is one of the advantages of treatment with plant-based cannabinoids, because of the ways they interfere with the body's ability to adapt to and overcome consistent treatment of any type. This consistency would hinder a treatment system that relies on nudging the body's out-of-balance systems back to balance. Medical cannabis does not block or replace the body's own systems of checks and balances; instead, it helps those systems to improve their abilities to restore equilibrium.

STRAINS

Cannabis is a prolific plant that can be grown anywhere. Where and how it is grown has significant effects on it and its phytocannabinoid and non-cannabinoid profile. One of the major divisions of the plant is between Cannabis *sativa* and Cannabis *indica*. These are the two major subspecies of cannabis, with many of their hybrids dominating local availability. Properties ascribed to the two subspecies are variable and largely inaccurate. As a rule of thumb, *Cannabis indica* is said to be more relaxing and focused on the body, making it a better choice for sleep and anxiety. *Cannabis sativa* is said to be more energizing and more of a cerebral "high," making it better while being active in one's life. However, these generalizations are inaccurate for any individual strain of the plant and any individual using it. Much is made of these differences, but there is no evidence for them other than a general sense among experienced users. Their experience, usually focused upon the effects of THC is quite different from inexperienced users and cannot be relied on to predict clinical response. Having stated this, there is some validity to the general claims, and a good place to start is to consider *Cannabis indica* for nighttime dosing for improved sleep and *Cannabis sativa* for daytime dosing of improved energy. How any individual will respond just isn't predictable. The best rule of thumb is to start either type of plant with small doses to gauge effects and increase slowly up or down as tolerated. This is especially true of hybrids of *indica* and *sativa*, which can vary in percentages of each component and make up by far the most numerous category of plant strains.

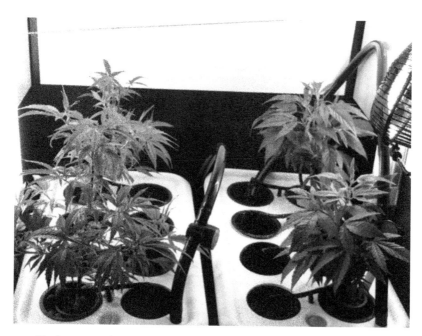

Early vegetative states of *Cannabis sativa* on the left and *Cannabis indica* on the right. Note the right's denser profile and broader leaves.

Far more relevant than these larger categories, is the actual phytocannabinoid profile of the individual plants. Here, truly infinite variability is possible, and we can come up with approaches that maximize this variability with the individual responses of each patient. Blending phytocannabinoids with the endocannabinoid system to enhance and improve our own built-in responses is the goal of treatment, determined by improvement of symptoms and actual physical signs. Sometimes these changes can be immediate, but these immediate responses often tend to be shorter-lived. More often the changes we are looking for are slower to occur and improve over time. Because the endocannabinoid system is so important for restoring balance to so many different systems in the body, slow progress is often rewarded with profound improvement. If the symptoms we are targeting involve persistent pain, the usual improvements start by reducing the size of the areas or body regions where pain is experienced, followed by decreased intensity of pain, then decreased flare-ups. Finally, abnormal persistent pain yields to normal acute pain related to pain-producing stimuli and a restoration of brain-based pain-processing circuits.

The body's endocannabinoid system has two jobs. Its first is to promote wellbeing, energy, and pleasure. Its second is to respond to specific injuries and insults to the body, by ramping up at the site of the damage to nudge the body back toward normal. Just as important, the endocannabinoid system and the phytocannabinoid system work at varied and deep levels in body and brain to re-establish this balance. This is relevant, because a slow rebalancing process is the norm for most chronic conditions helped by medical cannabis. That does not mean medical cannabis is not helpful for acute conditions or for reversing flare-ups of chronic conditions. It only means that the true gift of this treatment is in its ability to transform the body back to normal states in a slow, methodical way. This slow nudging back to normal is the best way to move from a state of disease to that of wellness, because it allows the body to slowly adapt to these changes to establish a new and lasting balance point of health and pleasure. Although some authors have speculated disease states as evidence of an endocannabinoid deficiency syndrome,[114] it is far more likely that the disease overwhelms these local systems, preventing it from restoring normal function. Rather than a deficiency of the endocannabinoid system, we should instead look at an imbalance caused by the injury or illness that needs some help to restore balance and normal function. Ideally, we could add a little anandamide (AEA) or provoke an increase of CB-1 or CB-2 receptors in local tissues, but there has been no clear clinical research on this approach, and too systemic and robust an increase in AEA or blockade of CB-1 or CB-2 receptors can be disastrous. Instead, phytocannabinoids augment the endocannabinoid system, then that

---

114   Russo EB. Cannabinoids in the management of difficult to treat pain. *Therapeutics and Clinical Risk Management* 4, no. 1 (2008): 245–259.

enhanced system boosts effectiveness of both the endocannabinoid and phytocannabinoid systems on brain and body. Since the systems interact so effectively and side effects are relatively benign or are even desirable, health promoting benefits far outweigh risks.

Exploiting the fact that CBDA is much more efficiently transformed to CBD by the body's metabolic processes than by heating it in an oven makes using raw cannabis an attractive idea. Almost all tinctures and edible cannabis products use extended heating of the plant to decarboxylate THCA, transforming it to THC. The same has been done to transform CBDA to CBD. The body does not decarboxylate THCA efficiently, but does decarboxylate CBDA. Blood levels of CBD up to 4 times higher with raw CBDA are attainable then with externally heated (decarboxylated) CBD.[115] Additionally, THCA and CBDA have their own powerful pharmacological effects and are not psychoactive. THCA is termed a mild euphoriant, but this is more likely related to its partial effects on brain CB-1 receptors causing a feeling of wellbeing and pleasure. Certainly, CBD has this effect indirectly by increasing anandamide availability and activity at CB-1 receptors. This opens up all types of possibilities of using the raw plant for a different therapeutic profile than the traditional use of the decarboxylated plant. Combining raw and heated plant to further pinpoint intended therapeutic action can also be an effective approach. It is also unclear what happens to the rest of the plant phytocannabinoids and other substances when heated. Studies need to be done and results published to determine what is clinically useful and what is not.

Specific plant strains are quite variable regarding phytocannabinoids and other components. They contribute to variation in physical properties (color, scent, flower structure, etc.), plant pharmacology, and effects on brain and body. Strains are bred for specific properties and are given specific names. Many of these names point to the breeding origins and hybrid nature of plants, but

---

115   Ujvary I, Hanus L, 90–101.

avoid the more formal Latin used in science. Instead a colorful and entertaining array of names are the rule: Purple Kush, Granddaddy Purple, Sour Diesel, Girl Scout Cookies, and Jack the Ripper. These strains are bred for various properties, most relating to the THC-based high, but high-CBD strains maintain this tradition, as well (AC/DC, Valentine X, Cannatonic, Harlequin, LT Fire, and Charlotte's Web). The variations of strains are nearly without limit, but local availability of any strain is a matter of popularity and suitability for growth in any given region. Different dispensaries contract with growers for the most popular brands for their clients. Alternatively, they may focus on specialty plants that are usually higher in CBD with contracted growers, or they may choose to grow their own.

Certain growers around the United States have focused on high-CBD plants. The accepted standard for a high-CBD plant is 4% CBD. This is a very liberal interpretation of "high CBD." Plants have developed and thrived with 25% CBD and above, and very low THC at less than 1%. Some have pursued these plant genetics to get truly high-CBD, low-THC cannabis plants, tinctures, and cannabis oil. The truth is that the whole spectrum of higher CBD plants is of great value, and these in combination and individually, preheated and raw, are quite useful medically.

A reliable and very informative website is Leafly.com. Leafly has a lot of information on many strains and keeps track of which dispensaries use specific strains in specific areas. It also has news and political sections that can be very informative, while promoting legalization and open discussion of recreational and medical use of cannabis. The caution with this website is with regards to specific medical benefits of specific strains. None of these have been studied, so what is presented is opinion. It doesn't mean that opinion is incorrect, but it isn't science, so take the specifics of it with a grain of salt. One area Leafly.com excels in is the reporting of scientific news and changes in the law. Another area is in actual descriptions of the ranges of various phytocannabinoids in different strains.

Rather than give a specific number, Leafly gives a range, which provides a ballpark figure for patients to explore local strains and their phytocannabinoid profile variability.

Although this part of the website is a good guide to availability where it states a strain is present, it can miss when it states a specific strain is not present. Most likely this is due to Leafly not having data from all dispensaries and looking only at flower or bud availability, not tincture and other embodiments.

It is important to reiterate that THC is a very useful and therapeutic cannabinoid, in and of itself. It is the phytocannabinoid that is most responsible for the high feeling many people seek, but it also exhibits anticarcinogenic, anti-proliferative, anti-inflammatory, antioxidant, analgesic, anti-anxiety, anti-epileptic, anti-nausea, anti-vomiting, neuroprotective, pleasure, and sleep-promoting effects.

Unlike alcohol, a nervous system poison, THC protects the nervous system and helps nerve cells resist degenerative conditions. Trying to avoid it removes a significant therapeutic tool from the cannabis arsenal. Timing its use to miss its high, if unwanted, is part of the art of medical cannabis treatment. High-THC cannabis can be consumed at bedtime. This promotes sleep and stress reduction, and if the person does not want to experience being high, they can sleep through it. If one does feel altered and wants to curtail that feeling, vaporizing a high-CBD, low-THC strain can quickly decrease and even eliminate the "high" feeling. This change occurs within minutes and is quite profound for most people. The sense of feeling cognitively altered is replaced with a general feeling of wellbeing. This does not work for everyone, and should be tested at non-critical times before relying on it in a socially important situation. This does not mean that this approach can be used to avoid a DUI or urine testing, as CBD does not lower THC levels. Rather, it alters psychotropic effects in a manner not yet understood. Once again, this is one of the main reasons that CBD was bred out of modern high-THC strains of marijuana.

Combining THC with high CBD, either through specific plant breeding or by mixing and matching several different plant strains, can be another effective way of limiting the high of THC. A plant with 10% CBD and 5% THC allows many people to avoid intoxication while smoking, vaporizing, or swallowing to ingest it. Mixing a plant that has 10% THC and little CBD with one that is 15% CBD with negligible THC can accomplish the same with higher levels of both. Again, individual variations are the rule, not the exception, and testing this before putting it to critical use remains important.

The truth is that no plant is high in either THC or CBD. They are actually high in THCA and CBDA until heated by smoking, vaporizing or preheating in an oven or on a stovetop. As previously stated, if the ingested plant matter is consumed without preheating, the body does not convert THCA to THC, but does convert CBDA to CBD. In fact, as previously stated, it converts CBDA at up to a four times higher amount than when the plant is preheated in an oven, vaporized or smoked. This phenomenon allows for a completely different therapeutic profile. A plant that is 15% THCA and 12% CBDA consumed without heat being applied will deliver virtually no THC, but provides high THCA, CBDA, and CBD levels. While CBD levels will take longer to peak, because they rely on the liver to transform CBDA to CBD metabolically, this also provides a longer time for it to be effective. Additionally, both THC and THCA break down to another active cannabinoid cannabinol (CBN). Thus, the therapeutic and side effects of THC are significantly decreased or eliminated with the above strain, but three other phytocannabinoid effects (THCA, CBDA, CBN) are added and increased, and CBDA transforms to CBD at up to a fourfold increase over the preheated plant. The whole idea of preheating comes from the practice of using heat to decarboxylate THCA to transform it to THC before being ingested, for intoxication. If, however, one wishes to avoid this or to consume THCA, CBDA, and CBN for their own medicinal effects, the raw plant offers new options.

TABLE 4: HEATED VS RAW PLANT

PHYTOCANNABINOID	HEATED	RAW
THC	Anti-cancer, anti-proliferative, anti and pro inflammatory, anti-oxidant, analgesic, anxiolytic and anxiogenic, anti-epileptic, anti-emetic (nausea and vomiting), neuroprotective, euphoriant, hedonic, sleep promoting	
THCA		Anti-spasmodic, anti-proliferative, anti-inflammatory, analgesic, pleasure, mild euphoria, well-being, anti-emetic (nausea and vomiting), neuroprotective

PHYTOCANNABINOID	HEATED	RAW
CBD	Anti-cancer, anti-proliferative, anti-emetic (nausea and vomiting), antibacterial, anti-diabetic, anti-psoriatic, anti-diarrheal, analgesic, bone stimulant, immunosuppressive, anti-ischemic, antispasmodic, vasorelaxant, neuroprotective, anti-epileptic, antipsychotic, anxiolytic	Anti-cancer, anti-proliferative, anti-emetic (nausea and vomiting), anti-inflammatory, antibacterial, anti-diabetic, anti-psoriatic, anti-diarrheal, analgesic, bone stimulant, immunosuppressive, anti-ischemic, antispasmodic, vasorelaxant, neuroprotective, anti-epileptic, antipsychotic, anxiolytic
CBDA		anti-proliferative, anti-emetic (nausea and vomiting), anti-inflammatory
CBN	Analgesic, anti-inflammatory, anti-cancer	Analgesic, anti-inflammatory, anti-cancer

Throwing in together different strains of cannabis, mixing different extractions, combining raw and heated strains, and shifting concentrations of all the phytocannabinoids provides an infinitely variable and constantly adjustable treatment strategy. While there is real appeal to being told how much of what to use, the constantly shifting endocannabinoid system is best optimized by a changing pattern of phytocannabinoid enhancement. Fortunately, this pattern is inherent in cannabis. Studies evaluating effectiveness of extraction of pure individual components clearly show that compared to the same amount of pure substance in whole plant extracts, isolated phytocannabinoids are not as effective.[116,117]

Once we start thinking about how to combine various phytocannabinoids in different ratios and blends, we can start considering compatible supplements and natural body processes to further adjust potential therapeutic benefits. In inflammatory conditions, raw high-CBDA cannabis ground up with curcumin is an interesting combination, with much potential as an anti-inflammatory. Combining CBD-dominant cannabis and curcumin presents intriguing possibilities, because both block nuclear factor kappa beta (NFKB), which is a major generator of inflammation and disease. The questions begging to be answered are the following: Would both substances working together to block NFKB have a more positive effect than either one separately? Would they cancel each other's effects out? Would their combined effects be additive, synergistic, ineffective or subtractive? The same can be asked about the combined effects of high-CBD cannabis with cayenne pepper. Both CBD and cayenne are potent blockers of the temperature sensitive receptor family. These both block the TRPV1 receptor that transforms acute pain to chronic pain and promotes bone loss

---

116 De Petrocellis L et al. Effects of cannabinoids and cannabinoid-enriched Cannabis extracts on TRP channels and endocannabinoid metabolic enzymes, 1479–1494.

117 Gallily R, Yekhtin Z, and Hanuš LO, 75-85.

in osteoporosis. Perhaps even more intriguing is the possibility of combining cannabis with other important substances the body produces to slow down the nervous system, stop and lower inflammation, and heal tissue, such as GABA, Interleukin-10 (IL-10) or Brain Derived Neurotrophic Factor (BDNF). Yet another possibility is to combine it with supplements like L-glutamine or vitamins such as methyl folate and methyl B-12.

Another good idea is to consider which symptoms are improved and which still need improvement, then augment current medical cannabis treatment with new approaches. An example of this would be if a person is using medical cannabis for pain and gets a positive result with a daytime high-CBD, low-THC strain, but continues to have sleep problems. Adding a higher-THC strain in the evening can significantly improve sleep. If THC causes anxiety or other unwanted issues, add some of the daytime high-CBD strain to it at bedtime to limit the psychotropic effects or change to a different more balanced strain. Other use, such as mixing different tinctures of different strains, can prove effective.

If tincture helps for sleep, but it takes too long to fall asleep, vaporizing a similar strain after taking the tincture may help begin sleep more quickly. This takes advantage of the rapid, short-lived increase of cannabinoids in the bloodstream with smoking or vaporization. Another example would be if using tincture during the day is inconvenient. In this case, ingesting tincture in the morning or evening and taking a capsule with a similar dose of the preheated, decarboxylated plant in the afternoon makes for a more convenient strategy. Furthermore, substituting the raw plant to achieve negligible THC absorption and metabolism, while providing anti-inflammatory, antispasmodic, neuroprotective, and analgesic effects of THCA is another approach that is less likely to cause an altered mental state.

Again, a word of caution is to try these approaches first when there is time to "sleep off" unwanted effects. Every person reacts differently to treatment with various strains of medical cannabis.

There is no standard "correct way" to use this treatment, and self-experimentation is extremely important to achieve positive outcomes. The idea of mixing medical cannabis with other supplements and the body's natural chemistry is appealing and is currently completely untested. Studies need to be designed to see if combining medical cannabis with other natural substances is beneficial and whether it offers any advantages over the plant or the substances alone. Use of raw plant material in capsules or other forms also points out the importance of testing raw cannabis to ensure it is clean of insecticides or other toxic substances.

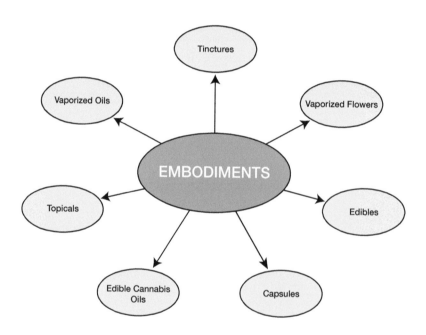

Next, we will review different embodiments of medical cannabis, including tinctures, topicals, vapor oils, edibles, flowers, capsules, and edible oils. Not only are there varied routes of administering cannabis available, but a balance of different plants and different preparations of those plants sculpts and refines this treatment.

TINCTURES

The whole plant is extracted from the flowers and leaves of cannabis to make the tincture. In this way, the ensemble effect of the plant is maintained. Having said this, the extraction process alters the plant's ratios of phytocannabinoids, and other substances and tinctures must be lab-tested to determine phytocannabinoid profiles. Tests of the plants that go into making the tinctures are not adequate. Tinctures of cannabis can be made in either alcohol or an edible oil, such as olive oil, coconut oil or safflower oil. Technically, tinctures are edibles, but they are so easy to titrate in small quantities that they deserve their own category.

Tinctures can be easily made at home, but are available at most medical cannabis dispensaries. There are numerous methods for making tinctures, and different tinctures can be mixed with each other to achieve a desirable result. While laboratory testing of tinctures will look at some of the major phytocannabinoids, most only look at THC and CBD values. Some do look at THCA, THCV , CBDA, CBDV, CBN, CBC, and CBG. Some recent measures include some of the more active non-cannabinoids found in cannabis, such as limone or beta-caryophyllene. Some labels describe concentrations as a percentage of phytocannabinoids compared to each other, mg/ml or number of mg per drop. All this is helpful, but because the ratios in the bottles change due to the passage of time, exposure to air and light, and variation of temperature, they are not totally reliable. Ultimately it all boils down to trial and error and educated guesswork. Practitioner and patient work together to refine this treatment, pinpointing symptoms and underlying conditions, while dialing in a wide variety of phytocannabinoids with similar and complementary properties. The use of tinctures makes this type of mixing and matching of various strains and their unique phytocannabinoid profiles a simple matter, without the health risk or social stigma of having to smoke or vaporize. One word of caution is that when mixing tinctures, mix only alcohol-based tinctures with other alcohol-based tinctures and oil-based tinctures with other oil-based tinctures, lest the combination of the alcohol and oil do not mix well. In the case of wanting to combine an alcohol with oil tincture, just take these separately.

Below is a typical titration schedule with a high-CBD low-THC tincture. Most patients well tolerate it, and it tends to minimize side effects.

Table 5: Titration of High CBD Low THC Medical Cannabis Tincture. Titrate at this rate if no unwanted psychoactive effects develop. If they do, lower the dose until there are none.

Day	Morning	Evening
Day 1	0 Drops	5 Drops
Day 2	0 Drops	10 Drops
Day 3	0 Drops	15 Drops
Day 4	0 Drops	20 Drops
Day 5	0 Drops	25 Drops
Day 6	0 Drops	30 Drops
Day 7	5 Drops	30 Drops
Day 8	10 Drops	30 Drops
Day 9	15 Drops	30 Drops
Day 10	20 Drops	30 Drops
Day 11	25 Drops	30 Drops
Day 12	30 Drops	30 Drops

Starting with a tincture makes this quite adjustable. Using high ratios of 18:1 to 26:1 CBD:THC, using 5 drops in the evening is a good starting point.

Five drops is an extremely low dose of both CBD and THC,

with the THC component being nearly negligible depending on the concentration of the tincture. This can be increased by five drops every day until reaching thirty drops. Then five drops can be added each day in the morning until the total of thirty drops twice daily is reached. Once there, this dose can be held for the rest of the month to gauge effects and side effects. No change in symptoms does not mean that the treatment is a failure, but instead indicates the usefulness of further upward dose adjustment (titration) and mixing and matching of different tinctures, while limiting the development of side effects.

The relatively high dose of CBD should cancel out any psychotropic effects at this dose, but this is not the experience of all patients. Some feel psychotropic effects at low doses. Psychotropic effects can be both undesirable and desirable:

Undesirable: Dizziness, dry mouth, forgetfulness, drowsiness, word finding difficulties, intellectual slowing, loss of motivation, psychological dependency, anxiety, paranoia

Desirable: Wellbeing, calm, positive mood, relaxation, stress reduction, euphoria, pleasure, happiness, enhanced taste, touch, vibration, scent, visual pleasure, sensual and sexual experience, and improved appetite.

Individuals have to decide the tolerability and enjoyment of these psychotropic effects. It is important to be able to minimize psychotropic effects for day-to-day situations, such as work, driving, and general performance of tasks.

One of the problems with any titration is that the relative concentration of the tincture varies. This means one drop of any tincture might be equal to two drops or more of another. Labels that give the total mg of CBD or THC are helpful, even though relative concentration changes over time. This will give an estimate of the concentration of phytocannabinoids of one tincture compared to another. At this point, labeling is not standardized, and until it is, labels should not be taken literally. As stated before, the changing phytocannabinoid ratios in all preparation of cannabis is desirable for medical purposes, due to the healthful properties of many of the phytocannabinoids and the theoretical impedance of the body's ability to adapt around the treatment.

An alternative to the above titration would be to start with one drop at night, and if no psychotropic effect occurs, then increase by two drops the second night, then two more drops the next night. If there are no psychotropic effects, then increase by five drops per night, as above. If this is too rapid an increase, then it can be slowed down. It is important to understand that this is an imprecise process because of the varied concentrations of the tinctures and the individual variation of the inborn endocannabinoid system in different people. This is the reason to always start low and at night, so that if undesired effects arise these can be resolved overnight, with sleep and the passage of time.

As stated earlier, learning how to use THC without feeling altered is an important goal. One way of doing this is to take a tincture at bedtime that is higher in THC, knowing that it will not take effect until one or two hours pass. Usually, the person is sleeping before feeling these effects. If sleep is problematic, a higher-strength THC tincture can be helpful. Most people familiar with cannabis will recommend a *Cannabis indica* plant for sleep, but this should be based on individual experience.

Table 6: CBD:THC ration 4:1 to 1:20 Titration Schedule

Day	Bedtime
Day 1	5 Drops
Day 2	10 Drops
Day 3	15 Drops
Day 4	20 Drops
Day 5	25 Drops
Day 6	30 Drops

30 drops roughly equals 1 milliliter (ml). Variation is accounted for by exposure to air, light, time, and temperature in the bottle. With alcohol-based tincture, evaporation is another issue and creates stronger tincture over time. This is recommended for use at bedtime, during titration. Sleep is usually improved and pain relieved within 60–90 minutes. Titrate according to your comfort level with the following psychotropic effects:

Negative: Dizziness, forgetfulness, drowsiness, word finding difficulties, intellectual slowing, loss of motivation.

Desirable: Wellbeing, calm, good mood, euphoria, pleasure, happiness, stimulation of body sensations.

Stop at the level with which you are comfortable. Feel free to go slower than five drops up or down at a time.

The above is a good place to start, using a high-CBD, low-THC tincture during the day and a higher THC tincture at night. There is nothing magical about a 4:1 ratio of CBD to THC or a 20:1 ratio of THC to CBD or anything in between. Instead, focus should be on what works for sleep and avoids THC's psychotropic effects in the morning, while benefiting from ongoing medical effects. Always start low, and if unwanted psychotropic effects do occur while increasing the dose, lower the amount and wait longer before titrating up again, if at all. If awakening with residual psychotropic hangover effects, taking the high-CBD tincture in the morning will usually cancel them out within 60–90 minutes. An alternative is to vaporize for a few puffs of high-CBD concentrated cannabis oil or plant that is very low in THC. This will usually clear the head at a much quicker pace of 3–5 minutes. As always, test this when there is time to wait out any unwanted psychotropic effects, in the evening or on the weekend. Some people will try to substitute edibles for this, but titration is much more difficult, and the amounts of THC stated on the packaging are rarely if ever accurate. The result can be an excessive amount of THC, causing anxiety, panic, and even hallucinations. Eating can also be problematic because the cannabis is not spread evenly throughout the edible, and any piece can be an overdose for any patient. Fortunately, as stated earlier, there is no lethal dose of cannabis, but unpleasant or unwanted side effects are to be avoided. Only experienced users should consider edibles, other than highly titratable and customizable tinctures or carefully selected homemade preheated or raw capsules.

There are many different types of tinctures, and they can be mixed and matched. Again, it is important to remember that if using an oil-based tincture and mixing tinctures together, do so with another oil-based tincture. Alcohol tinctures can also be mixed together for more varied results. One can mix and match both, but they should be consumed separately. Alcohol-based tinctures are best diluted in an ounce or more of water or juice to dilute the 150 to 190 proof alcohol used to make them. This stops the burning sensation in mouth and stomach when consumed. This also masks any unpleasant flavor and can certainly be further diluted if desired. Sublingual absorption does not return a particularly high blood level and is unnecessary.[118]

Leaving a tincture under the tongue for 20 minutes makes some logical sense, but this does not necessarily translate into higher or quicker absorption rates and is impractical for many. Blood levels of cannabis can be deceiving, with uptake into brain, liver, kidney, lungs, and fatty tissue being predictably higher in tissue than in blood.[119] While oral absorption is challenging, it delivers a low blood-level and high tissue distributions with extended periods of activity. It is also a good idea to use the oil-based tincture if maintaining sobriety. While cannabis is not a gateway drug, alcohol certainly is one. Even this small amount of alcohol is best to avoid if one has a history of alcohol abuse or is taking Antabuse.

Regardless of whether a tincture is made with alcohol or edible oil,

---

118   Ujvary I, Hanus L, 90–101.

119   Heustis MA. Human Cannabinoid Pharmacokinetics. *Chemistry and Biodiversity* 4, no. 8 (2007): 1770–1804.

it is almost always made from preheated cannabis to decarboxylate THCA and CBDA into THC and CBD. This is a tradition that arises from recreational use of cannabis. THCA does not alter the vast majority of individuals psychologically or cognitively. The problem is that some degree of heat is inherent in the preparation with oil, making it highly likely that significant amounts of THCA will be converted to THC. Although alcohol doesn't need to be heated, the extraction of what is in the plant, using this method, can still activate some of the THCA to THC. Up-to-date testing is important to determine relative ratios of substances, but should not be relied on for accuracy over the period from testing to consumption.

Some commercially prepared tinctures are actually combinations of several different strains of plants. These can be done to change the phytocannabinoid profiles to reflect more balanced treatment approaches, but claims of specific therapeutic effects should only be used as a guideline. Individual results are highly variable. People tend to believe what is written on labels, but remember that the labels on preparations of medical cannabis are not particularly accurate, especially claims that certain strains or preparations are disease-specific. Experimenting with different tinctures and combinations of tinctures can help against acute symptoms.

Most chronic illnesses need to be evaluated over a period of weeks to months, not hours. This includes chronic inflammation and its associated illnesses. Since most chronic illnesses are either caused by or create chronic inflammation, this is a very important clinical way that medical cannabis may help with disease states from diabetic cardiomyopathy to degenerative conditions of the nervous and connective tissue and various forms of cancer.

VAPORIZATION AND SMOKED

Patients are just as likely as most physicians to believe that medical cannabis involves smoking a joint. While smoking cannabis can be an effective treatment approach, most consider vaporizing a healthier alternative. This approach involves the heating of the plant or related concentrated oil-based plant extractions to a temperature that decarboxylates THCA and CBDA to THC and CBD, but does not burn the plant. Instead, a water-based vapor containing the phytocannabinoids is inhaled and expelled. Most importantly, this eliminates most of the tars associated with smoking. There are no credible studies that show harm from inhaling cannabis smoke, but this does not mean there is no harm. An occasional smoked cannabis cigarette or pipe is not likely to be harmful, but vaporizing is a good alternative that is less of a theoretical risk than smoking cannabis, especially with regular medicinal use.

One compelling reason for medical cannabis to be legalized is that it would be much easier to use in other inhaled devices, such as inhalers or discus delivery systems. In fact, recently an Israeli company, Syqe, has developed a device that allows inhalation of cannabis. It has licensed the device to the largest generic pharmaceutical company in the world, Teva, to bring to market. This device has been tested for a year by Haifa's Rambam Health Care Campus, with approval of the Israeli Health Ministry. Investors include the Phillip Morris Corporation. This development promises to bring medical cannabis to patients without the need to smoke or vaporize the plant, using extracted plant granules, otherwise unaltered, in measured dosing. A small study done with this device showed blood levels at 3 minutes below expected vaporized levels at an average of 38 ng/dl plus or minus 10 ng/dl, with greater uniformity, lower side effects (light-headedness), and 45% pain reduction. The pain relief peaked in twenty minutes and lasted an average of 90 minutes.[120]

---

120   Eisenberg E, Ogintz M, Almog S. The pharmacokinetics, efficacy, safety, and ease of use of a novel portable metered-dose cannabis inhaler in patients with chronic neuropathic pain: a phase 1a study. *Journal of Pain and Palliative Care Pharmacotherapy* 28, no. 3 (2014): 216-225.

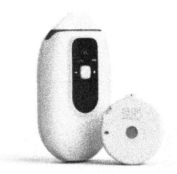

Perhaps the most significant thing about all this is the mainstreaming of botanical delivery in a true medical device. Medical cannabis treatment has developed without organized medicine and Big Pharma backing it, and yet here are the premier generic company in the world and deep-pocket investors, working with a cannabis-focused startup to bring a safe delivery device and extraction technique to qualified patients. Furthermore, the Israeli government fully supports this. Here is the real shocker. The premier Israeli researcher, Raphael Mechoulam, has had full and unbiased support for his research from funding from the United States National Institute of Health. He has gone on record to state that the NIH never tried to have any influence on the type of research he did or its outcome, a very different situation than our government-sponsored medical cannabis research in the United States.

Starting with the whole plant is a more time consuming and less convenient method than using concentrated cannabis oil, but it has the benefit of being the whole, unadulterated plant. No extraction or concentration process has been applied here, only heat. This activates several of the natural acid forms of the plant to their decarboxylated forms. Hence, not only are THCA and CBDA transformed to THC and CBD, but THCVA is transformed to THCV, CBGA to CBG, etc.

Traditionally, smoking the whole plant has been the way people have used cannabis for millennia. This has proven a reliable way to get decarboxylated phytocannabinoids into the body (mainly THC) quickly and efficiently, but it also loses the advantage of delivering the acid forms of phytocannabinoids, which can have their own medicinal properties. This is a reason why the best medicinal strategy for most people is to use tinctures (mostly decarboxylated), vaporized plant or oil (decarboxylated), and oral capsules (carboxylated), combined. This presents the broadest phytocannabinoid profile to the body. If this can be done with different strains it adds to the rich variability of therapeutic and synergistic substances.

EDIBLES

Edibles are foods with cannabis cooked in. The problems with edibles make them a poor choice for patients who are inexperienced or avoidant of psychotropic effects. They are too unpredictable in effect, and impairments can last quite a long while. They tend to be high-THC oriented, although high-CBD products are available.

They are often cooked into appealing and delicious preparations, such as cookies, brownies, chocolate bars, sucking candies, and gummy bears. This promotes overconsumption, and is an attractive looking treat to children to sneak and eat. As with all medical cannabis treatments, they need to be kept secure from children in an inaccessible, locked storage area. Psychotropic effects can become hallucinatory and paranoia-inducing with this form of consumption and variables of tolerance, metabolic rate, individual genetics, and elimination add to the unpredictability of this approach to treatment. If one does decide to try this treatment, reading the label (despite notorious labeling inaccuracies) with a focus on testing and ratios of phytocannabinoids can be a helpful guide. This is best used before sleep the night before a day off work or responsibilities, so that if unwanted effects do occur, there will usually be adequate time for them to clear before having to deal with day-to-day tasks. I would not recommend edibles (other than tincture) for anyone who is uncomfortable with the psychotropic effects of cannabis. Even when a label describes high CBD and low THC, care should be taken by starting with 25% or less of the recommended dose.

One other way to approach this is with capsules of ground-up plant, either raw or preheated or a combination of both. These also can be titrated, but ideally tried after using a tincture from the same plant, if available. A capsule of decarboxylated (heated) or carboxylated (raw) cannabis is a more convenient way of using this treatment, but is also to be approached by experienced users only. Some dispensaries sell capsules with decarboxylated plant or concentrated oil in the capsule. Both can be effective treatment. People can make their own capsules by purchasing "00" or "0" size gelatin empty capsules at health food stores or on line and filling them with ground-up plant. The "0" capsule is easier to swallow for many and is the better choice in general. Capsules afford a relatively constant amount of cannabis to use in a neat and convenient package. This also allows the user to vary the contents of the capsule for more precisely directed, highly variable treatment options. Ingesting capsules can also be a more cost-effective way of getting treatment, especially if a person grows their own cannabis. This is another reason why obtaining or growing only organically grown, pesticide-free, uncontaminated cannabis is important.

The original cannabis concentrates involve pressure with or without heat to the resin glands of cannabis flowers. If no heat is used, this is called kief, and if low heat is applied, it is known as hashish or hash. While this can be ingested, the results are often unexpected, as a lot of hashish already has converted THCA to THC by the pressure and heating technique. It is very hard, if not impossible, to find available high-CBD, low-THC hashish or kief in medical cannabis dispensaries. If one is growing high-CBD cannabis plants, this can be made at home. The paraphernalia chapter will give details on this.

Concentrated cannabis oil, often inappropriately named hash oil (unless it is made from hashish), is usually dispensed in syringes with marked measurements, to be consumed orally in very small quantities. The oil itself can have waxes in it or the waxes can be removed. It can also be delivered as shatter, which is caramelized or flakey texture of cannabis oil. These tend to be very high in concentrations of THC and/or CBD, hence much less is needed to attain desirable effects or unwanted side effects. Shatter is usually smoked or vaporized, but can be consumed orally in very small quantities.

One advantage of concentrated cannabis oil is that once the desirable quantity is determined, it can be delivered into small size 2 or 3 capsules. This makes for a more portable treatment that can be carried around and used more discreetly than pulling out a syringe and dispensing it onto the finger. It also eliminates the unpleasant, bitter taste of this embodiment of medical cannabis. The best of these concentrated oils are made with a cold CO_2 extraction process or are made by gently evaporating off the alcohol in a 95% alcohol base, then adding a small amount of olive oil to reconstitute the residue into an edible oil base.

Cannabis oil can also be used as a vaporized or dabbed concentrate to inhale. Vaporizing has the advantage of fewer tars than dabbing, which entails placing a drop of concentrated cannabis shatter or oil on a titanium bar called a nail, applying a flame heat source, and inhaling.

TOPICALS

Largely because of lack of safety restrictions of the plant, lack of regulation by the FDA, and the irrepressible spirit of human ingenuity, wildly variable preparations have appeared to improve on medical cannabis. Topical treatment is often available in limited form in various dispensaries. These are made in specific balms and lotions, with baseline inactive ingredients ranging from various commercially available lotions to more customized underlying composition. Beeswax is often used as a thickening agent. These preparations tend to be high in THC, but high-CBD products are available.

It is harder to find the high-CBD topicals then it is to find high-THC products, but THC is very unlikely to cause any systemic or psychotropic effect in this form. Sometimes topicals are unscented, but this often leads to an individual smelling like cannabis when they rub this on and for some time thereafter. Other times, these are scented with various products, usually essential oils, which can lead to rather delightful scented preparations. These topical products are pleasing to touch and smell, while providing immediate, regionally specific relief without systemic effects. When essential oils, such as peppermint, lavender, or tangerine are added, the inherent properties of these essential oils (analgesic, anti-inflammatory, anti-microbial, etc.) can also contribute to symptom improvement, disease relief, health, and wellness. In neuroplastic approaches to pain, we use scent and touch quite freely to counter-stimulate the brain pain circuit's constantly firing and expanding pain map. All senses can be used to help decrease pain in the present and train the brain to restore normal pain responses, with touch and scent as particularly accessible and useful counter-stimulating sensory experiences. Topical cannabis preparations with a pleasing scent, soothing and positive stimulation of touch receptors, and analgesic and anti-inflammatory effects can be profoundly helpful. Some patients use topical treatment with outstanding and immediate results. Adding a few drops of cannabis tincture to any topically applied treatment (even those that already contain cannabinoids) can allow these patients to customize their own treatment. Here, adding various combinations of tinctures can help to figure out which topicals work best for which problems, developing deeply customized approaches to treatment, and augmenting and using already helpful therapeutic topicals. The likelihood of any unwanted psychotropic effects is negligible with this type of embodiment.

ROUTES OF ADMINISTRATION

Again, human ingenuity knows no bounds. Preparations have been developed that include the above, plus soaps, shampoos, leave-in conditioners, suppositories, edibles of every type, entire meals cooked with cannabis, cannabis oil heated and inhaled on a titanium nail, phytocannabinoid crystals, cannabis-infused olive oil for cooking or salads. The spectrum of available products is only limited by routes of access to the body. These include oral, inhaled, rectal, vaginal, topical, transdermal, transbuccal (cheeks and gums), and sublingual (beneath the tongue) approaches. In scientific experimental treatments, even intravenous and intramuscular injectable forms have been developed and used. Doubtless, if there is some way to get cannabis into the body, someone has tried it.

Soaps can be made incorporating medical cannabis oil-based tinctures. This infuses them with the phytocannabinoids in the tincture. The skin contains massive amounts of cannabinoid receptors on nerve endings and in the skin's dermal layer as part of the inflammatory and anti-inflammatory systems. A soap containing cannabinoids followed by a body lotion also containing them can be very helpful to reduce a systemic rash's itching and pain, by blocking inflammation. Topical cannabis treatment may also prove itself to be quite helpful in treating precancerous skin lesions and even skin cancers themselves, but more study needs to be done to figure out which combinations of phytocannabinoids are most helpful. Using tincture directly applied to the skin can help with pain even deep below the surface.

Shampoos introduce another use of oil-based cannabis tincture with shampoo to treat scalp-based inflammatory disease. This includes seborrhea (dandruff); itching, burning, and painful scalp rashes; and scalp-based pain from inflammation, headaches, and trigeminal neuralgia. Following the shampoo with cannabis infused leave-in hair conditioner can leave a film of cannabis on the scalp for more lasting effects. Headaches in general, migraines, and trigeminal neuralgia facial pain inflamed nerves of the scalp, which feeds back on the headache pain and makes it worse. In the same fashion, getting control of the scalp-based pain feeds back on the deep structures of the brain that keep headaches going, and can go a long way to reducing them. Using soap-making formulas or adding oil-based cannabis tincture to commercially available shampoos, leave-in conditioners, and emollient, commercially available lotions can result in extremely pleasant substances, with appropriate scents that can be helpful with rashes, pain disorders, and itching.

PHASES OF TREATMENT WITH MEDICAL CANNABIS

Treatment phases can be categorized as beginning, intermediate, and advanced. Particular characteristics distinguish each phase of treatment.

Beginning treatment is about finding out which strain and embodiments are best tolerated, while addressing the condition one is trying to control. Is it inflammatory, stress, pain, neurodestructive, cancer-related, sleep-related? This phase is also about measuring initial responses to the substances used to determine what to try next. Is the course of treatment causing cognitive impairment? Intermediate treatment is about expanding the Total Cannabinoid Profile (TCP) to present a more varied stimulus to the endocannabinoid system and the numerous non-cannabinoid systems. Phytocannabinoids then work in combination on these enhanced systems involved in restoring mechanisms of balance, and push the body toward health and wellbeing. This is brought to further fruition in the advanced phase of treatment, in which phytocannabinoids are constantly varied and phytocannabinoid and supplementary non-cannabinoids are combined to prevent body processes from adapting and circumventing these effects. The goal of either curing chronic illness or rendering it dormant is an important aspect of this advanced stage of treatment, and the broad, varied, and rotating TCP increases the chance of this by preventing brain and body from figuring out a way around this treatment. This is a particularly encouraging aspect of medical cannabis-based treatments, because one of the problems with traditional treatment with pharmaceuticals is the body's tendency to adapt and adjust over time.

Phases of Care

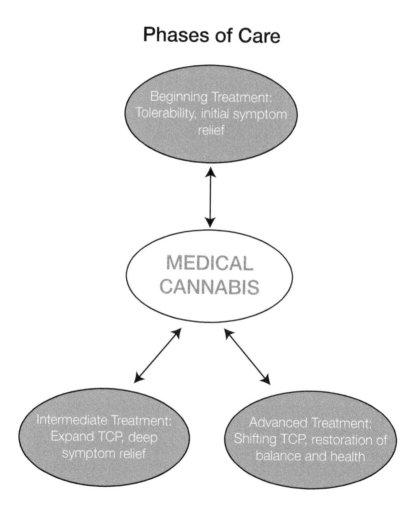

TCp= Total Cannabinoid Profile

BEGINNING TREATMENT

Tinctures are an excellent way to start treatment, because they are so easy to titrate. Although five drops in the evening is a good place to start, some people will want to start at one drop and go up one drop at a time instead of five drops. This is fine. The goal of beginning treatment is to find out what works, but also what is tolerable and how much is needed for symptom relief and restoration of health. The treatment must fit the patient's life, not the other way around. Although we can figure out how to use this treatment with almost everyone, without psychotropic effects, the road to achieving this requires tolerance of these effects to determine dosing limits. Rarely, some people are unable to tolerate either the olive oil or alcohol used in tinctures. In these cases, there are ways to slowly increase cannabis in other forms or embodiments. Still tinctures remain quite flexible. One distinguishing factor of medical cannabis from recreational cannabis is more varied use of the different forms, phytocannabinoid profiles, and convenience of use in both private and public situations. Tinctures fit well with aspects of each of these factors. They come in different forms (alcohol or oil), and concentrations can be varied by their preparation and, in the case of alcohol-based forms, evaporation. They are easy and quick to use and consume discreetly. Additionally, they are widely varied and can be mixed for even more variety.

Tinctures are particularly useful for beginning treatment, even for experienced recreational users, because they shift emphasis from psychotropic effects to medical benefits. This helps people develop an underlying profile of use that stays focused on health benefits and away from being psychotropically or cognitively altered. Once again, if people enjoy being "high" using THC, they can still use a high-THC form of the plant when convenient. They can also learn how to use cannabis to help their particular condition while remaining in normal consciousness. This is not to say that tinctures lack psychotropic effects. These can actually be quite profound, but because of their slow onset, they can be used to advantage to help with sleep or sexual function. More importantly certain tinctures can be used during the day, without any psychotropic effect on the user. This is particularly helpful for developing around the clock therapeutic levels of non-psychotropic aspects of medical cannabis. The development of therapy that does not impair is the constant goal of medical cannabis treatment. Desirable psychotropic effects can be added, if and when patients decide these would be useful. In this way, unwanted psychotropic effects can usually be avoided.

Most chronic conditions are variable and involve acute periods when the condition is worse and better. In the cases of pain and mood disturbances, these variations usually result in increases and decreases of symptoms. In more silent underlying disorders, such as cancer, hypertension, and organ deterioration, symptoms may be subtler. In these cases, worsening problems may present with general fatigue, not feeling well, or development of new symptoms. Medical cannabis tinctures can help decrease acute symptoms, but their real strength is in nuanced, less immediately obvious benefits of decreasing the contributions to illness of the underlying condition. More immediate benefit to acute symptoms can often be achieved by adding vaporization of concentrated cannabis oil or cannabis flowers into the established treatment with tinctures. It is helpful to develop a routine of using tinctures first to establish a safe and effective baseline treatment. Then vaporization can be added to bring persistent or worsening symptoms under control quickly. Vaporization of cannabis is of almost immediate benefit, when compared to tincture. In the beginning stages of medical cannabis treatment, vaporizing cannabis oil with a special vaporization pen is easy and quite convenient. Vaporization of cannabis is not a very long-lasting treatment, because of the much more rapid metabolism of the phytocannabinoids. These do provide an immediate and rather high blood level, with a rapid peak at 90 seconds to 5 minutes, rapid tissue distribution, and elimination from tissue in up to 2–4 hours. The beauty of adding this approach to the longer-lasting, lower-blood-level, higher-tissue-level treatment of orally ingested cannabis is in being able to use it effectively for acute symptom or symptom breakthrough management. Vaporizing cannabis oil can determine if new symptoms, feelings of illness, and feelings of fatigue respond to more rapidly increased blood and tissue levels. In a sense, this can become the touch-up treatment for bothersome short- and long-term worsening of illness. Once a sense is established of how any individual does with particular tinctures, vaporization of similar strains of cannabis oils can be used. In general, using the same vaporized cannabis oil as the tinctures will be more predictable of psychotropic effects and help the individual patient determine what is effective, while maintaining safety and freedom of use. Having said this, it is still advantageous to rotate to different strains, regardless of embodiment.

TABLE 7: BEGINNING MEDICAL CANNABIS TREATMENT

Embodiment	CBD:THC Ratio	Titration	Psychotropic Effects
Tincture	18:1–26:1– During the Day	5 drops or less gradually increased to 30 drops in AM and Afternoon	None expected
	4:1 to 1:1 At Bedtime Use an Indica tincture if possible (not critical)	5 drops or less gradually increased for good sleep and no hangover	Yes–Increase as ratio shifts toward higher THC, will occur while asleep

TABLE 7: BEGINNING MEDICAL CANNABIS TREATMENT(cont'd.)

Embodiment	CBD:THC Ratio	Titration	Psychotropic Effects
Vaporized	Use 20:1 to 26:1 During day and start with trying this at night	1 vape, then wait 3 minutes and try again. May keep doing this	None expected
	Use 4:1 to 1:1 at Bedtime	1-2 vapes wait 3 minutes. This should cause drowsiness. May use more	Yes–Effects are immediate. Light headed, euphoric, well-being, dizzy, drowsy

INTERMEDIATE TREATMENT

Combining embodiments, routes of administration, and timing of treatment builds on beginning treatment that is best accomplished with titratable tinctures and expanded to use of vaporized concentrated cannabis oils. Once this treatment is established and routines are developed, introduction of more varied use of tinctures, vaporized oil, topical, transdermal, and edibles can be combined with preheated and raw plant and vaporized or smoked cannabis flowers. The idea in this phase of treatment is to increase the TCP, with treatment outcome expectation of deepening symptom relief. Vaporizing concentrated cannabis oil is simple, but using the raw plant, while more complicated, provides the widest phytocannabinoid and terpenoid profile for immediate availability. Sometimes it is easier to find a raw plant that has the desired combinations than it is to find specific tinctures or cannabis oil. Every embodiment of medical cannabis starts with the raw plant. This also provides more do-it-yourself types of options. For those who enjoy preparing their own food, clothing, and customized projects, using the raw plant as a launching pad for more creative treatment establishes both an attractive option and a satisfying and pleasurable activity. Additionally, it is in starting with the plant and openness to self-experimentation that symptom and disease management can be pinpointed, augmented, and refined.

Capsules can be filled with cannabis in the raw (carboxylated) or preheated (decarboxylated) form. To clarify this, cannabis plants contain the precursors of many phytocannabinoids, not just CBD and THC in their acid forms. These include THCA, CBDA, THCVA, CBCA, and others. It was thought these forms were inactive, but that was based on the notion that the only considered activity of cannabis was its psychotropic effects. As we have learned more about the medicinal value of the plant and have studied the phytocannabinoid components that contribute to it, it has become clear that the acid forms of phytocannabinoids have many important therapeutic properties of their own. A capsule made of finely ground, unheated cannabis of any type is unlikely to cause psychotropic effects.

Some THCA is converted to THC in the drying process known as curing the plant, and testing in a safe time and place is always an option. Usually the amount of THCA transforming to THC by the curing process is negligible, but some people are highly sensitive and should take a test dose first. THCA can cause a feeling of calm and wellbeing on its own that might feel to some like a psychotropic side-effect, but likely this is about anxiety reduction and not being cognitively impaired. The metabolic pathway in the body for THCA does not break it down to THC, but instead makes CBN, another non-psychoactive phytocannabinoid, with analgesic, anti-inflammatory, and anticarcinogenic effects. THC also breaks down to CBN, so imbibing the raw plant or heated plant both result in development of a CBN level. This use of decarboxylated (heated) or carboxylated (raw) plant or both at the same time expands options.

Table 4 shows that treatment with preheated and raw cannabis from the same plant can be quite different. One can also see that consumption of both raw and heated cannabis in varying ratios to each other can provide even more blended and variable treatment.

Titration of capsules is a process that allows for an increase in dosing in a methodical way to find the best effects. This can be accomplished in several ways. Empty gelatin capsules can be purchased in variable sizes from the small number 3 capsules to the large 00 ones. One can start with a small size and, depending on side effects, can increase this to larger sizes. Another approach is to pick a "0" or "00" capsule and only fill it 1/4 full, then add more cannabis to each subsequent dose, until the capsule is full or side effects ensue.

TABLE 8: INTERMEDIATE MEDICAL CANNABIS TREATMENT

Embodiment	CBD:THC Ratio	Titration	Psychotropic Effects
Vaporized	18:1 to 24:1 During the day 1:1 to 1:20 Bedtime	Two dropper's full in morning and late afternoon	None
	1:1 to 1:20 Bedtime	One–two dropper's full	Yes–while sleeping
Vaporization– Oil or Plant	20:1 to 26:1 during day AC/ DC, Valentine X, Remedy, Charlotte's Web	Vape 8-12 times over 15 to 20 minutes	None
Vaporization– Oil or Plant	2:1 to 1:20 In evening and bedtime Omrita Rx, Harlequin, Cannatonic, LT Fire Blackberry Kush, Blue Dream	Vape 4-12 times to help fall asleep	Yes–before sleep or earlier in evening if preferred, if being altered is desirable
Capsules– Cooked	24:1 to 26:1 Pre-heated in oven 300° for one hour AC/DC, Valentine X	1. Increasing capsule size 2. Fill a quarter of a "0" capsule and increase amount slowly	None
Capsule–Raw	Any strain. CBDA:THCA ration is same as given CBD:THC ratio	1. Increasing capsule size 2. Fill a quarter of a "0" capsule and increase amount slowly	None, but test in safe time

The above table can be used as a guide for intermediate treatment. Remember, different people experience medical cannabis in different ways, due to the wide variability of our own ever-changing endocannabinoid system, personal genetic variations, and unexpected changes in plant phytocannabinoid profiles. Always test a new treatment out during safe times. Even experienced users can have unexpected psychotropic effects, so a little care is indicated, especially when changing treatment. Get to know individual strains, both raw and preheated.

Tinctures can transform THCA to THC by the process with which they are made. Raw plant matter that is ground up and put into capsules is dramatically different in effects from the preheated plant in capsules or smoked and vaporized flowers. Figuring this out for a particular condition can be quite rewarding.

Advanced Treatment

The hallmark of the advanced phase of medical cannabis treatment is the rotation of strains and embodiments, to present a constant, but ever-shifting cornucopia of phytocannabinoids, routes of administration and supplementation. Sculpting treatment by balancing phytocannabinoids, terpenoids, and other plant-based substances takes an already sophisticated treatment approach to new levels of customization and augmentation. The advanced treatment phase underpinning is that of finding a stable and broad set of treatments and rotating them throughout the day and between each day. This interferes with brain and body finding work-arounds to medical cannabis treatment, as they so effectively do with many other forms of treatment. While the plant changes itself over time, this active shifting of phytocannabinoids is a more substantial and guided way of delivering a changing but stable treatment. This treatment phase can also include exposing the plant to something that purposefully alters it in a specific, directed fashion (light, heat, oxygen, time), as well as combining it with non-cannabinoid and neuroplastic treatments.

Multiple strategies can be employed. The simplest approach is to mix and match different strains of cannabis and count on Mother Nature to sort out phytocannabinoids for you. This is a very reasonable strategy that does require some planning and thoughtfulness. First and foremost, a decision about whether a person wishes to be mentally altered should always be the starting-off point. If this is desired, vaporizing a high-THC, low-CBD strain is a good way to begin. This can be followed by using a tincture with 1:1 CBD. If there is a desire to limit the length of psychotropic effects of cannabis, then adding a 20:1 to 26:1 vaporized high-CBD:THC plant will likely take the high down over the next 15 to 30 minutes. This may not completely resolve these effects and should be tested, as always, in non-critical time. If, on the other hand, one wishes to not be altered, then a tincture or capsule of high-CBD:THC cannabis is the way to begin. This can be followed with vaporizing a different high-CBD:THC strain, rapidly raising CBD blood levels with the vaporized strain and keeping high tissue levels with the orally ingested strain. The reason to select different strains is due to varying phytocannabinoid profiles other than just CBD and THC.

Preheating one strain and mixing it with a raw similar or varied strain can also dramatically change the phytocannabinoid profile. If using a heated and raw version of the same plant and putting this combination in capsules, slowly build it up. Capsules are highly recommended because they are so portable and convenient. Heating a plant that is high in CBD and mixing it 1:1 in with a plant that is high in THCA, THCVA, or CBDA can deliver a completely different ratio of phytocannabinoids. There are plants that when vaporized or smoked will leave the user significantly altered and impaired but have no such effect when ingested in a capsule. It is best to consider that all tinctures are made with preheated plant material, as that is the overwhelming tradition. If it is stated that this is not the case, it is worth having it independently tested if possible before using, to get a clear phytocannabinoid profile at the time of the testing. Even this will change in the future, but likely keep a similar ratio. Again, this can be tested over time by a reliable laboratory to see if it is so.

Another choice is to let cannabis with a high THCA content sit out in light and air to transform much of it to CBN. Test it for THC, THCA, CBD, CBDA, and CBN at the beginning of this approach and over time (try 6 months to a year). Recreational cannabis users would consider this exposure to light and oxygen a sure way to degrade the plant, but if the goal is to avoid higher THC-related psychotropic effects, this can be yet another strategy for altering the plant to get more desirable treatment profiles and options. Likely this effects the breakdown of other phytocannabinoids as well. It should be tested to get a broader idea of what is changing.

Mixing raw or preheated plant with raw cacao powder, curcumin, and/or cayenne pepper can augment various interactions of the phytocannabinoid system with the body's endocannabinoid, vanilloid, and immune systems. As stated earlier, raw cacao contains anandamide, one of the body's endocannabinoid neurotransmitters, an anti-inflammatory. In fact, raw cacao has over 100 times more anandamide than the chocolate in various candies and baked items, which is roasted at 480° for 24 hours, cooking away most of the anandamide and the enzymes that keep it active for longer. The phytocannabinoid CBD has many actions in the body, but one of its most important properties is to increase the availability of anandamide by preventing it from being broken down. Logically, it makes sense to add a food such as raw cacao, that not only contains anandamide, but also has agents in it that prevent anandamide from being degraded. Curcumine (Turmeric) is a prominent spice used in Indian food as the major ingredient in curry. It is anti-inflammatory, blocking NFKB, a signaling molecule at the core of all the inflammatory cascades. CBD blocks many of these cascades, but is also a strong blocker of NFKB. The combination presents interesting possibilities for profound and deep alteration of chronic inflammatory problems, which are at the root of almost all chronic conditions, leading to the gradual deterioration of the human body and most illness-related deaths. Cayenne pepper in combination with medical cannabis also presents interesting strategies. Cayenne pepper, THC, CBD, CBC, CBN, THCA, CBDA, CBGV, THCV, CBN all stimulate and desensitize the family of vanilloid receptors (TRPV-1, TRPV-2, TRPA-1, TRPM-8). This appears to result in an anti-inflammatory, anticarcinogenic effect. Furthermore, anandamide (increased by CBD and raw cacao) also stimulates the TRPV-1 receptor, opposing inflammation, chronic pain, and bone loss.[121] Thus adding cayenne pepper to cannabis capsules is another way to potentially inhibit inflammation, pain, and cancer. While all this needs to be studied further, an interesting combination of raw and preheated cannabis, raw cacao, turmeric, and cayenne pepper present a potentially potent cocktail of plant-based herbal treatment to fight inflammation, cancer, and chronic pain. While there is no evidence that any of this could cure these conditions, they could go a long way toward helping people with any or all these problems to have healthier and better lives.

---

121   De Petrocellis L et al. Effects of cannabinoids and cannabinoid-enriched Cannabis extracts on TRP channels and endocannabinoid metabolic enzymes, 1479–1494.

TABLE 9: ADVANCED TREATMENT

Embodiment	CBD:THC Ratio	Titration	Psychotropic Effects
Tinctures	18:1 to 24:1 During the day	Three dropper's full in morning and late afternoon	None
	1:16 to 1:20 Ratio at Bedtime	One–two dropper's full	Yes–while sleeping
Vaporization– Oil or Plant	20:1 to 26:1 during day (examples: AC/ DC, Valentine X, Remedy, Charlotte's Web)	Vape 8-12 times over 5 to 10 minutes	None
Vaporization– Oil or Plant	1:1 to 1:20 In evening and bedtime (examples: Bubba Kush CBD, Critical Cure CBD, Blackberry Kush, Blue Dream)	Vape 4-12 times to help fall asleep	Yes–before sleep or earlier in evening if preferred
Capsules– Cooked	20:1 to 26:1 Pre-heated in oven 300° for one hour AC/DC, Valentine X, Remedy	"0" or 00"capsule Fill whole capsule	None
Capsule–Raw	Any strain. CBDA:THCA ration is same as given CBD:THC ratio	"0" or 00"capsule Fill whole capsule	None, but test in safe time

The rotation of these treatments results in a broad phytocannabinoid profile. A typical weekly treatment would involve the following (strain names are given as an example to illustrate the rotation of strains, to broaden and vary the Total Cannabinoid Profile (TCP):

TABLE 10: ADVANCED TREAMTENT—WEEKLY ROTATION

Day of Week	Morning	Afternoon	Evening	Bedtime
MON	High CBD AC/DC Tincture 90 drops (24:1) Pre-heated High CBD Electra Capsule (10:1) Vaporize High CBD Remedy	Pre-heated High CBD Ringo's Gift Capsule (22:1) Pre-heated High CBD plus Raw High THCA Capsule (2 strains)	Vaporize 24:1 to 1:1 CBD:THC No high to mild high	1:20 Indica CBD:THC Tincture plus 1:20 variable Vape
TUES	High CBD Valentine X Tincture 90 drops (25:1) Raw High THCA Capsule (1:20) Vaporize High CBD Therapy	Pre-heated High CBD Electra Capsule (22:1) Raw High THCA capsule (1:20) (2 strains)	Vaporize 10:1 to 1:1 CBD:THC No high to mild high	1:20 Indica CBD:THC Tincture plus 1:20 variable Vape

Day of Week	Morning	Afternoon	Evening	Bedtime
WED	High CBD Remedy Tincture 90 drops (24:1) Pre-heated High CBD plus Raw High THCA Capsule (Four strain) Vaporize High CBD AC/DC	Pre-heated High CBD Valentine Capsule (25:1) Raw High THCA capsule (1:20) (3 strains)	Vaporize 4:1 to 1:20 CBD:THC Mild high to high	1:20 Indica CBD:THC Tincture plus 1:20 variable Vape
THURS	High CBD Ringo's Gift Tincture 90 drops 22:1) Pre-heated High CBD plus Raw High THCA Capsule (Two strain) Vaporize High CBD Valentine	Pre-heated High CBD Charlottes Web Capsule (22:1) Raw High THCA capsule (1:20) (4 strains)	Vaporize 29:1 to 1:8 CBD:THC No high to high	1:20 Indica CBD:THC Tincture plus 1:20 variable Vape

Day of Week	Morning	Afternoon	Evening	Bedtime
FRI	High CBD Therapy Tincture 90 drops (24:1) Pre-heated High CBD Ringo's Gift Capsule (22:1) Vaporize Combo of M-Th	Pre-heated High CBD AC/DC Capsule (24:1) Raw High THCA capsule (1:20) (5 strains)	Vaporize 7:1 to 1:20 CBD:Mild high to high	1:20 Indica CBD:THC Tincture plus 1:20 variable Vape
SAT	High CBD Electra Tincture 90 drops (10:1) Pre-heated High CBD Therapy Capsule (22:1) Vaporize High CBD Two strain	Pre-heated High CBD Therapy Capsule (22:1) Raw High THCA capsule (1:20) (3 strains)	Vaporize 22:1 to 7:1 CBD:THC No high to mild high	1:20 Indica CBD:THC Tincture plus 1:20 variable Vape

Day of Week	Morning	Afternoon	Evening	Bedtime
SUN	High CBD Charlotte's Web Tincture 25:1) Raw High THCA capsule (Five strain) Vaporize High CBD Five Strain	Pre-heated High CBD Remedy Capsule (24:1) Raw High THCA capsule (1:20) (2 strains)	Vaporize 24:1 to 1:3 CBD:THC No high to mild high	1:20 Indica CBD:THC Tincture plus 1:20 variable Vape

This type of approach not only quite broadens the TCP, but delivers a constantly variable profile to the body. This can include more than twenty different strains, four different embodiments (tincture, capsules, vaporized oil, vaporized flowers), and preheated versus raw flowers. Of course, this can be made more variable or less. Regardless, this should make it much more difficult for the body to adapt to the treatment.

This approach should eliminate the sense of being cognitively altered or high during the day, but allow for this in the evening if preferred. If a person has difficulty with even the smallest amount of THC, substituting 20:1 or above CBD:THC preparations for the higher THC preparations or using raw plant with high THCA should eliminate any high. Again, the caution is to try this out during a safe time before introducing this during the day. Weekends can also be a time for experimenting and substituting higher THC strains and embodiments. This can be tried with less fear about psychotropic effects, although not for those who are uncomfortable with THC effects.

As stated earlier, medical cannabis is a neuroplastic treatment. This means that the treatment alters the nervous system, promoting new and varied connections; neurotransmitter introduction, modification, and utilization; receptor stimulation; and blockade; genetic changes; brain-based anti-inflammatory responses; and birth and deployment of new nerve cells. The literature is full of studies that show these effects with both the endocannabinoid and phytocannabinoid systems.[122,123,124] Neuroplastic change is a very active process that results in over 7.5 out of 1,000 trillion synapses changing in the adult human brain every week.[125] This means that new connections are made and broken at this astounding rate. Since the phytocannabinoid system works well with the endocannabinoid system, we have a treatment capable of shifting brain structure and function in a positive direction to change chronic disease states to balanced states of wellbeing, energy, and pleasure.

Cannabis and GABA (gamma-Aminobutyric acid) are yet another interesting therapeutic combination. GABA is the body's own main inhibitory neurotransmitter. Its job is to turn off nerves that are firing too frequently, while leaving those that are firing normally alone. It is the second most common neurotransmitter in the brain and the most common in the entire body. GABA is instrumental in shutting off nerve pain, stopping anxiety, and inducing the resting state rhythms of the brain, among many other modulating functions throughout the body. Taking this with medical cannabis high in THC or THCA leads to greater results than the mere additive effects of the combination. Using this combination to help with sleep is yet another intriguing possibility.

L-glutamine, which more readily crosses the blood-brain

122   Chiuchiu V, Leuti A, Maccarroni MJ, 268-280.

123   Aguado T, 1551–1561.

124   Walter C et al., 1659–1669.

125   Stettler DD et al. Axons and Synaptic Boutons Are Highly Dynamic in Adult Visual Cortex. *Neuron* 49 (2006): 877–887.

barrier than GABA, but is transformed to GABA once it does so, is another option. The table below shows the effects of combining raw or preheated plant material with raw cacao (high in anandamide), turmeric (potent anti-inflammatory through blockade of NFKB), cayenne (transforms chronic pain to acute by stimulation of TRPV-1 receptors), and GABA (the main inhibitory neurotransmitter in the body).

TABLE 11: USING CAPSULES TO CONTROL PSYCHOTROPIC EFFECTS

Embodiment	Combination	Psychotropic Effects
Capsules	Raw + cooked high CBD plant	No
	Raw plant + Raw cacao	Possible–strain dependent
	Cooked plant + Raw cacao	Possible–strain dependent
	Cooked +Raw plant + raw cacao	Possible–strain dependent
	Raw plant + Tumeric	No
	Cooked plant + Tumeric	Possible–strain dependent
	Cooked +Raw plant + Tumeric	Possible–strain dependent
	Raw plant + Cayenne	No
	Cooked plant + Cayenne	Possible–strain dependent
	Cooked +Raw plant + Cayenne	Possible–strain dependent
	Raw plant + GABA	No
	Cooked plant + GABA	Possible–strain dependent
	Cooked + Raw plant + GABA	Possible–strain dependent

As stated earlier in this chapter, we can use tinctures to add cannabis to any topical agent. By doing this, the topical treatment can be highly customized. The risk of any psychotropic effects with this are infinitesimally low. This way, THC can be added to topical treatment for people that struggle with this treatment systemically. Additionally, phytocannabinoid profiles can be greatly expanded by mixing several tinctures into topical treatment.

TABLE 12: COMBINED CANNABINOID TREATMENT

Embodiment	Combination	Psychotropic Effects
Tincture	1. CBD:THC >15:1 2. CBD:THC>1:1<15:1 3. CBD:THC >1:24<1:1	1. Slow, high CBD and very low THC levels with slow onset and vast high tissue levels. Works within 1-2 hours and lasts 8 hours 2. Slow, moderate CBD and THC levels with slow onset and vast high tissue levels. Works within 1-2 hours and lasts 8 hours 3. Slow, low to moderate and high THC levels with slow onset and vast high tissue levels. Works within 1-2 hours and lasts 8 hours
Vaporized Oil	1. CBD:THC >20:1 2. CBD:THC>1:1 <20:1 3. CBD:THC >1:24 <1:1	1. Rapid, high CBD and low THC levels with quick onset and moderate tissue levels. Works within 1-3 minutes and lasts 3 hours 2. Rapid, moderate CBD and THC levels with quick onset and moderate tissue levels. Works within 1-3 minutes and lasts 3 hours 3. Rapid, low to moderate CBD and high THC levels with quick onset and moderate tissue levels. Works within 1-3 minutes and lasts 3 hours

Embodiment	Combination	Psychotropic Effects
Vaporized Plant	1. CBD:THC >20:1 2. CBD:THC>1:1 <4:1 3. CBD:THC >1:24 <1:1	1. Rapid, high CBD and low THC levels with quick onset and moderate tissue levels. Works within 1-3 minutes and lasts 3 hours 2. Rapid, moderate CBD and THC levels with quick onset and moderate tissue levels. Works within 1-3 minutes and lasts 3 hours 3. Rapid, low to moderate CBD and high THC levels with quick onset and moderate tissue levels. Works within 1-3 minutes and lasts 3 hours
Capsule	1. CBD:THC >20:1 2. CBD:THC>1:1 <20:1 3. CBD:THC >1:24 <1:1	1. Slow, high CBD and very low THC levels with slow onset and high tissue levels. Works within 1-2 hours and lasts 8 hours 2. Slow, moderate CBD and THC levels with slow onset and high tissue levels. Works within 1-2 hours and lasts 8 hours 3. Slow, low to moderate CBD and high THC levels with slow onset and high tissue levels. Works within 1-2 hours and lasts 8 hours

Embodiment	Combination	Psychotropic Effects
Topical	4. CBD:THC >20:1 5. CBD:THC>1:1 <20:1 6. CBD:THC >1:24 <1:1	1. Rapid, high CBD and low THC levels with quick onset and high local and low systemic tissue levels. Works within 1-3 minutes and lasts 2-4 hours 2. Rapid, moderate CBD and THC levels with quick onset and high local and low systemic tissue levels. Works within 1-3 minutes and lasts 2-4 hours 3. Rapid, low CBD and high THC levels with quick onset and high local and low systemic tissue levels. Works within 1-3 minutes and lasts 2-4 hours

This sophisticated treatment is a long way from lighting up a joint and getting stoned. It reflects the absolute lack of limitation of medical cannabis treatment. It promotes self-exploration, best done in concert with one's physician or another knowledgeable practitioner. By varying embodiments, delivery systems, plant strains, and decarboxylation, one can drill down the granular nature of this treatment to the deepest levels of the human body. Because cannabis is so safe relative to all prescribed drugs and almost all over-the-counter drugs, while being a potentially robust treatment for some of the worst conditions affecting people, excellent treatment outcomes can be achieved with minimal side effects and safe use. One can enhance that safety by using strains and embodiments that do not result in being impaired. Also, avoiding inherently unsafe activities if psychotropically altered is not only a socially responsible way to use this treatment, but an essential one if this it is to remain available in states where it has been legalized for medical use.

Following 140 cases in my practice for an average time of twelve months, I noted the following improvement:

1. Improved Pain   84.1% (116/137) 2.2% (3/138) Worse

2. Improved Stress   72.1% (101/140) 0.7% (1/140) Worse

3. Improved Sleep   81.4% (114/140) 0.7% (1/140) Worse

4. Improved Quality
    of Life   75.5% (105/139) 0.7% (1/139) Worse

5. Improved Energy   53.2% (74/139) 7.9% (11/139) Worse

6. Improved Focus   42.4% (59/139) 7.2% (10/139) Worse

7. Opioid Reduction   68.7% (73/111) 7.2% (8/111) Stopped

These numbers are remarkable. Different types of cannabis were used regarding embodiment, strain, and routes of administration. All treatment was customized to each patient, and all were using some other type of medication concomitantly. Perhaps the most extraordinary figure is that 68.7% of people using opioids to treat their chronic pain reduced their opioid use. All these patients had serious pain disorders, most having sustained severe injuries, including low back degeneration, cervical spine degeneration, neuropathic pain, inflammatory pain, and/or central nervous system pain. 111 of the 138 were on opioid medications, and more than two-thirds (73) reduced this during the period they were followed. These were not forced or even recommended reductions, except that we let people know that several people had been able to reduce their medications using cannabis. Still, 68.7% of these patients reduced their opioids voluntarily, without structured direction or program. That is an observation of major importance, because of the safety issues involving opioid treatment of persistent pain. Perhaps an even more important finding was the astonishing number of people who reported pain relief and the high correlation with people reducing their opioids. Most were taking both CBD and THC dominant preparations. Many were in the intermediate stage of treatment.

Specific recommendations were made as to what to try at a specific dispensary, and instructions for use were emailed to the patients. Patients were encouraged to text with any problems or concerns, and these were answered, usually by the next day, with recommended dose, strain, and embodiment adjustments.

CASE STUDIES

LS is a 65-year-old woman with a history of migraines several times a week, sometimes lasting for days to weeks, since age 18 (47 years). This is complicated by degeneration of her cervical spine and emergency neurosurgery 10 years ago for a bruise that developed on her spinal cord after an epidural block. She also has aching body pain. Her headaches worsened after the neurosurgery, but she was already disabled from them prior to this procedure. She is very sensitive to medications and has not done well with anti-inflammatories, nerve pain medications, antidepressants, and muscle relaxants. She has had some benefit from opioid medications and benzodiazepines. Medical cannabis was started 2 months ago with a high-CBD low-THC tincture (26:1), and she slowly increased this to 30 drops twice daily. At this point she could abort a building migraine in an hour. No medication or combination of medication had done this in the past. Subsequent return of migraines prompted further upward adjustments to 60 drops twice daily. This gave her a week without migraines. When a strong migraine returned, we increased this to 60 drops three times daily, and migraine was completely abolished for the next month. The only side effect is daytime sleepiness, which was present before starting medical cannabis, but is worse on it. She has steadily lowered her opioids and benzodiazepines.

GS is a 41-year-old woman who has been using medical cannabis for a severe and disabling anxiety disorder following abuse of her prescribed amphetamines and abuse of alcohol two years ago. She has a long-standing history of anxiety and obsessive-compulsive disorder. She has burning mouth syndrome, probably secondary to nicotine and alcohol use. She has improved sleep, stress, quality of life and focus after 11 months of slow upward titration, punctuated by periods of abstinence from medical cannabis due to monetary concerns. She now is using 60 drops of high-CBD, low-THC cannabis at night, vaporizes 2–4 puffs at a time during the day, and uses tincture of the AC/DC as needed during the day. She does not have relief of her burning mouth, but this is a minor problem. She has stopped drinking and has returned to work as a hospice nurse administrator.

LS II is a 29-year-old patient with Ehlers-Danlos Syndrome, an underlying disorder of collagen formation that leads to multiple signs and symptoms, including spontaneous joint dislocation, deterioration of biological barriers, histamine release and reactions, severe alterations of the autonomic nervous system, massive food sensitivities, excessive inflammation, and severe pain. She learned and utilized a general approach using neuroplastic transformation techniques to rein in her pain. Adding medical cannabis has been immensely helpful, especially vaporizing high-CBD strains, including LA Confidential, AC/DC, and Valentine X. As is the case with most people with her variation of this disorder, sensitivity to drug side effects is the rule, not the exception, and even therapeutically effective treatment can become problematic over time. Additionally, effects that are the opposite of usual medication activity are common. Using medical cannabis has resulted in markedly decreased food sensitivities, joint dislocations, and pain flare-ups. She is much more robust and much more functional. Baseline pain remains significant at times, but is no longer constant. She can reduce pain and anxiety when either is present.

AB is a 65-year-old woman who becomes anxious with use of THC. She has had chronic low back pain, which has made it difficult for her to travel even a few miles by car. She started with a 24:1 tincture and gradually added other strains, including a higher 4:1 CBD:THC tincture, and stopped the morphine she had been taking for over 20 years.

DB is a 64-year-old woman who has had complex regional pain syndrome (CRPS) for several years. She stopped morphine, which she had taken for the severe pain associated with her condition, by using tinctures, preheated 24:1 CBD:THC capsules, raw capsules that were 1:1 CBDA:THCA, and vaped higher THC cannabis concentrates at night. She is relatively pain-free most of the time.

Chapter 5

Dispensaries

HERE IN NORTHERN CALIFORNIA, THERE is an extremely small medical cannabis dispensary run by a visionary genius dedicated to relieving the suffering of people. He has 4,000 patients in his dispensary, which is certainly considered to be a small operation. To put this in perspective, most urban dispensaries in the state have tens of thousands of patients or more and the largest dispensary has over 110,000. He has organically grown and developed over thirteen high-CBD plant strains, with six strains at 20:1 to 25:1 CBD to THC. He has many others with different percentages of CBD:THC ranging from approximately 3:1 to 1:3. He makes tinctures and concentrated cannabis oil out of them. He blends the tinctures and oils, combining them to achieve different ratios of phytocannabinoids. He also grows high-THC plants that he also makes into tinctures and oils. He is constantly experimenting to improve his strains. He does not sell his brand to other dispensaries and carefully tests his plants in all the embodiments he makes. He treats his plants as "sacred medicine," and his wife sings to and blesses them daily with a beautiful Hawaiian hula ceremony as they grow. He uses the most sophisticated scientific approaches to growing these plants and puts his patients' needs above his own. His motivation is helping others rather than making money. He constantly updates and refines his products and works on ways to use medical cannabis without people being altered unless they wish to. He reads the scientific literature about medical cannabis and figures out how to incorporate new findings with what he grows and how he makes various embodiments. He attends cannabis conferences and contests and stays focused on producing the most medically valuable plants and products. He is open to new ideas and willing to try the things that make sense to him. He talks to the patients who are members of his dispensary about their problems, and comes up with individualized approaches that work through any issues they might be having. He is kind to everyone. He knows he is doing what he is supposed to do.

He is writing a book about CBD. What he knows must be passed on to a younger generation of growers who are focused on high-THC plants for recreational use, to help them understand that growing high-CBD plants that do not make the user high will always be in demand for medical cannabis treatment. He knows that for this treatment to grow and thrive, the public perception of medical cannabis users being stoned all the time must shift to an understanding of the usefulness of medical cannabis to help people remain highly functional and involved in their lives. Most importantly, he knows that he has helped many people to transform serious illness and despair to wellness and hope.

This is one of the four basic models of medical cannabis dispensary. Since laws are different in each state, and administered differently at the level of counties and towns, there are massive variations of these dispensary models available. They tend to fall under four basic models that I have called *farm to medicine cabinet, co-op, boutique,* and *department store models.* As medical and recreational cannabis are approved in state after state, these models vary, but remain the basic four models of the vast majority of dispensaries. There are advantages and drawbacks to each, and these need to be understood to achieve the best outcome in selecting treatment options.

It is important to recall that the variations in this treatment are truly infinite, and that this is one of the strengths of this approach to care. As care advances, availing oneself of the variation of treatment can make a difference. One of the hard things for novice users of these dispensaries is the discomfort involved in going to a dispensary and navigating the experience. Experienced users must set aside the idea that if they do not feel altered, the medicine is not working. It helps the patient to be informed and to have a basic understanding of his or her needs, so that he or she, rather than the dispensary, determines the treatment. This chapter will not only look at the specific models of dispensaries, but will also address other topics, such as the way that products are displayed, online ordering, dispensary-based research opportunities, membership, and the art of informed choice.

FARM TO MEDICINE CABINET DISPENSARY

The dispensary described at the beginning of this chapter represents one of the four basic medical cannabis dispensary models. All have many positive attributes and some drawbacks. I call this model of care the *farm to medicine cabinet* model of dispensary. This involves a small operation owned and operated by a skilled cultivator. Embodiments are made by hand, testing regularly to assure quality and relative accuracy of labeling. Business is focused on a high percentage of CBD-based products. This type of dispensary also sells high-THC products, but recognizes the need for balance that goes beyond CBD and THC ratios. These small operations can produce high quality, organically grown plants or work with small organic farmers who grow for them. They carefully select indoor and outdoor growing methods that are ecologically sound. Selection of high-CBD products can exceed those of much larger dispensaries.

These are reliable dispensaries whose products can be trusted by both patient and treating physician. The focus in this type of dispensary is decidedly medical.

Embodiments are made at the dispensary and individually tested after being made. From growth to embodiment, no poisonous pesticides are used and totally organic approaches are employed.

On the downside, their overall stock is often limited compared to the larger operations. Although prices may be higher, quite often they are competitive. They may even be lower than at larger dispensaries. The choices of high-THC plants are often less than at larger dispensaries, and products are less varied. High-CBD plants and embodiments often sell for more than those that are high in THC.

The real advantage of this model is the proprietor's meticulous care and knowledge of the products being produced and sold. The proprietor not only has an excellent understanding of the strains produced, but also has close relationships with any other growers or producers they may use. Their products are often handmade, never mass-produced or grown. The plants are well tended and testing is usually extensive, with more custom information available. These growers recognize the variability of phytocannabinoid and terpenoid profiles from strain to strain and even plant to plant. Often, the farm to medicine cabinet model of dispensary will provide clones, care, and growing instructions that are invaluable when patients are trying to save money and grow their own plants. The personal touch available at a dispensary of this type often goes beyond the budtender or salesperson, and extends all the way to the owner. The owners of the dispensary are extremely knowledgeable about their own plants and embodiments, and are frequently a fountain of knowledge about other strains, dispensaries, and growers. Often if a patient has a request for the owners to grow a different strain, they will research it and, if they can locate seeds or clones, will try growing it to make it available for sale. These growers do tend to specialize in rare and exotic plants with unusual profiles, and this can lead to interesting pharmacological properties.

Because of the personal touch in this type of dispensary, it is a good place to start care. It is far more difficult to find, but searching can be worth the effort. Patients can let their physicians know about such dispensaries, and knowledgeable physicians can direct their patients to them to be able to recommend appropriate plants and expect reliable results. Another advantage of this type of dispensary is the maintenance of consistency of products.

THE CO-OP MODEL

The *co-op model* is similar to the farm to medicine cabinet model in the way it involves personal care by co-op members, but consists of members growing their own plants. These usually require a restricted number of members coming together to designate one as the grower for the other members. This type of dispensary usually can only sell to their own members. Records must be kept by a designated member of the co-op. Grows are usually organic, but may incorporate non-organic techniques, depending on the decision of the members. Their greatest advantage is that prices tend to be quite good, because of the way all members contribute to the finances, work, and function of the co-op. There are also more informal but similar models in some states and areas. These aren't dispensaries, but involve a designated grower for a group of patients with medical cannabis licenses and designated growing for the members only. These do not require the record-keeping of the other models, but involve self-policing to make sure all members are certified and have assigned growing rights to the grower. These grows are often labors of love, and involve a lot of personal care and attention. Grows in medical cooperatives are usually high in CBD, but also have higher-

THC plants available. The plant number restrictions determine the variety of plant strains.

The problem with this model is that it is quite limited. The quality of the grow will depend on the knowledge and experience of the grower. Depending on the size of the co-op and state and county restrictions, products other than the raw plant may or may not be available, and everything is usually less formal and less standards-driven. Trimming, presentation, and sales are far more informal than in the other models, although this is not always the case. The effectiveness of the co-op model requires dedication and devoted members.

These types of dispensaries are also a good place to start care. A co-op should grow a variety of plants for best results: those very high in CBD and very low in THC, and those high in THC and low in CBD. Additionally, it should make much more than the flowers available to members. All the leaves trimmed from the plant before and after harvest should be saved for juicing or use in salads or smoothies to benefit from the fresh and raw aspects of the plant. Alternatively, making cannabis concentrates from the leaves is an effective use of what is often thrown away. It is always a good idea to test the plant to understand the phytocannabinoid and terpenoid profiles. This gives excellent information in more advanced phases of treatment, when these profiles can be mixed and matched together during the day to deliver more complete and effective care. In this model, everyone is taking care of everyone else. This allows for very specific plants to be grown, not only to meet any co-op member's needs, but also for the overall good of the group. It also allows for making embodiments most desired by the members.

This model is skewed toward people with serious medical disorders, because it is the seriousness of medical problems that leads co-op model members to be dedicated.

THE BOUTIQUE MODEL

The hallmark of this model is a small storefront that contracts with growers, transporters, and manufacturers to procure its products. It caters to clients in a relatively small space with a broad product range. These dispensaries are usually highly secure with state-of-the-art monitoring systems, security guards, and well-organized patterns of moving people through their lines. These tend to be short in general, but can build up over peak times on weekends and evenings.

People can see the various products on display, and helpful staff is full of useful information about the plant varieties. If an individual budtender does not know the properties of a strain, they can call in a supervisor who will. These dispensaries tend to know their growers and have a large enough group of them that they are always receiving new products. They do their own trimming of the plants they receive. Frequently, they have a doctor on premises who can evaluate and certify the patient. These physicians are quite knowledgeable and will help patients understand the basics of treatment. They usually have various clones available for people to grow their own cannabis. These *boutique-model* dispensaries have some paraphernalia available, but it is usually limited due to space constraints. The websites of boutique-model dispensaries are often a little quirky, but online purchases for members are usually clear and well organized. Pictures of products are professionally and beautifully done. Recent boutique dispensaries have been very high-end, with smoking and vaping rooms, much like the smoke rooms in high-end tobacconist shops. There will often be a budtender available to make suggestions and even offer tastings. These high-end dispensaries are quite plush and cater to people who appreciate gourmet products and services. While limited, all their products are of the highest quality, while fetching the highest prices.

On the negative side, boutique dispensaries tend to emphasize high-THC cannabis, which has its place, but is no substitute for a balanced phytocannabinoid profile, using high CBD and low THC during the day. The number of high-CBD, low-THC products in these boutique dispensaries tends to be limited, and usually they pair fairly high amounts of THC with most high-CBD products they do stock. There is nothing wrong with these products, but the high-CBD, high-THC products tend to cause significant psychotropic effects. Novice users need to be careful when using these. Online descriptions of product effects tend to be rather subjective, but can be used as a general guide. While physicians may be available on premises for certification, follow-up treatment is not part of the dispensary routine. Patients can sometimes arrange for follow-up visits, but this is not available as a routine part of treatment in most boutique dispensaries.

Insurance does not pay for patient care or certification, but this is true of all dispensaries. Quality of plants and embodiments tends to be excellent, but prices are often quite high. The consumer, when comparing prices, should be careful to determine equivalent amounts between dispensaries, as some sell half the size as others for the same or higher price. Paraphernalia is not extensive, but what is present tends to be of high quality. The very high-end boutique dispensaries tend to charge a premium that can be double or triple that of regular boutique dispensaries.

The boutique model of dispensary is a good dispensary for people who know what they need. It gives a broad range of choices with little to no wait. The presentation of the products is usually excellent, and the budtenders tend to know a lot about the plants. Knowing what you are looking for is a better idea than just asking advice.

That doesn't mean that asking advice is not helpful. It is just best done from a position of knowledge than of ignorance. For the consumer, looking for a close-matching phytocannabinoid profile is usually a better idea than seeking a specific species.

THE DEPARTMENT STORE MODEL

The *department store model* of medical cannabis dispensary is just what it sounds like. These tend to have vast inventories and services that go beyond just selling products. Often, they have lectures and discussions from knowledgeable people in the medical cannabis field. They will have groups that meet for various issues, from using cannabis for harm reduction from other drugs and substances to groups that meet to discuss the needs of the community. They will also provide contracts for growers and, because of the vast size of their clientele, can certify qualified growers to grow all or part of their plants for the dispensary. This provides the grower a safety-net document that certifies them as growing for the patients who are dispensary members. The product inventory tends to be vast, and department- store-model dispensaries will often provide for special orders. Owners of these large dispensaries are usually quite politically active and well connected. These dispensaries provide employment with good benefits to their employees, and can be some of the area's largest employers, even in large urban centers. They pay local taxes and follow the medical cannabis laws meticulously, to make sure that their businesses can tolerate scrutiny of regulators and law enforcement. They have effective attorneys backing them up, and will often fight excessive regulation and law enforcement, with a good record of winning these conflicts in court. Their websites are highly professional and product choices are vast. This includes various medical cannabis strains in every type of embodiment. Their use of vendors and manufacturers tends to be of high quality, and price structure is built around supply and demand. Because of the huge number of members in these operations, buying power is excellent. Storefronts are usually quite large and varied, with vast displays of products and other activities being put on throughout the space. Products can be found at these dispensaries that are not available anywhere else.

On the downside, the sheer volume of products is often quite overwhelming and intimidating to the novice user, especially the older adult. Some medical advice is neither accurate or consistent, but employees are usually very compassionate and helpful. Lines and waiting times can be long and inconvenient. These places have varied CBD plants and products, but like the boutique dispensary, tend to have higher amounts of THC. These dispensaries have vendors from all over their state. Quality control is important, but as in any big operation, mass production of products can be problematic at times.

These department store model dispensaries are true community resources. Again, they are best approached by those who know what they want. While they may not have the exact strain being requested, the budtenders are very helpful in pointing out similar plants. These larger dispensaries usually have more varied paraphernalia choices and a knowledgeable staff. Beyond the help available to individual patients, these dispensaries tend to be the most involved with federal, state, and local regulations and politics. They become important economic engines in their communities, benefitting those areas and the state. Choice, dispensary buying power, political savvy, cannabis-based special interest groups, and cannabis education help make these dispensaries much more than just a buying experience for those interested. These dispensaries also have doctors available for evaluation and limited treatment. They also keep referral sources of physicians who practice cannabis-based medical treatment.

In summary, there are four basic models of medical cannabis dispensaries. They all have advantages and drawbacks. If a person is lucky enough to live in an area with all four models, they should try each type to see which fits best for them. Beginners with cannabis in general and medical cannabis specifically should try the farm to medicine cabinet or co-op to start treatment, if possible. Part of my purpose in writing this book, however, is to make any of these dispensaries less intimidating and more useful by providing detailed information about the treatment and ways to look at this as a changing process. One type of a dispensary or another may prove to be more useful, depending on what a person is looking to add to their treatment regime. Remembering to vary phytocannabinoids and using strains, embodiments, delivery systems, and carboxylated/decarboxylated plants provides a rich profile of phytocannabinoids that make it difficult for the body to work around. Varying models of dispensaries may be necessary to fill this need, as treatment becomes more familiar and complex. It is important to remember that the human brain places high priority on both familiarity and novelty. A stable but thoughtfully changing system of phytocannabinoids presented to and beyond the endocannabinoid system can help deliver effective long-term treatment.

TABLE 13: MEDICAL CANNABIS DISPENSARY MODELS

Dispensary Model	Advantages	Drawbacks
Farm to Medicine Cabinet	Small, master grower, organic, hand made embodiments, regular testing, high CBD, low THC specialization, highest quality, thoughtful advice, personal touch, consistency, organic Good Place to Start and Stay	Smaller Selection, harder to find, may or may not have higher prices, little or no available paraphernalia, high CBD plants may be more expensive
Cooperative	Lower prices, member chosen plant strains, member involvement in all aspects of the co-op, more than just flowers available for greater variety of uses by members, everyone looks out for everyone else Good Place to Start	Potentially less consistent, may or may not be organic, small selection, little or no available paraphernalia, quality depends on ability of grower(s)

Dispensary Model	Advantages	Drawbacks
Boutique	Good variety in store and on-line, plants from trusted sources, attractive displays of products, rapid transit through the purchase process, limited paraphernalia, may have a doctor on premises or on referral, high end products and settings available, some high end "destination" dispensaries are available Best if you know what you need	Can be overwhelming to novice users, tend to emphasize high THC products, high CBD products are often also high THC, packaging overstates specificity of product effects, absent or very limited follow up treatment from on premises physicians
Department Store	Largest variety in store and on-line, broadest variety of plants and embodiments, attractive displays of products, good supply of varied paraphernalia, usually have doctor on premises, Best if you know what you need	Can be overwhelming to novice users, tend to emphasize high THC products, high CBD products are often also high THC, may have very long lines, packaging overstates specificity of product effects, absent or very limited follow up treatment from on premises physicians

Joining a Medical Cannabis Dispensary

In the United States, different states have different regulations, and it is beyond the scope of this chapter to lay each one out specifically. NORML, the National Organization for the Reform of Marijuana Laws, has a listing of state cannabis laws for each state at the following web address http://norml.org/laws/ , which reviews individual state regulations. A subsequent chapter about the law will go into greater detail. The states that do have medical cannabis laws vary. At this writing, only six states in the US do not have some form of medical cannabis. Several states have CBD-specific laws. These are often quite restrictive regarding medical condition, physician role, embodiment, possession limits, and cannabis availability. The following states have CBD-specific medical cannabis laws:

> Alabama Florida Georgia Iowa Kentucky Mississippi
> Missouri North Carolina Oklahoma South Carolina
> Tennessee Texas Utah Virginia Wisconsin Wyoming

NORML describes the Texas law as nonfunctional. This is because it requires physicians to write a specific prescription, which would put them on the wrong side of the federal law. All other states stick with the standard practice of physicians providing certification for treatment, rather than a specific prescription.

These states have less restrictive medical cannabis laws, but vary in their details:

> Alaska Arizona Arkansas California Colorado
> Connecticut Delaware District of Columbia Hawaii
> Illinois Louisiana Maine Maryland Massachusetts
> Michigan Minnesota Montana Nevada New
> Hampshire New Jersey New Mexico New York North
> Dakota Ohio Oregon Pennsylvania Rhode Island
> Vermont Washington

In total, forty-four states and the District of Columbia have some form of medical cannabis laws. Thirteen out of sixteen CBD-only states do not allow for state sponsored dispensaries. Only four out of twenty-nine states with medical cannabis laws do not have state-sponsored dispensaries, but several programs are not yet functional. Each of the twenty-eight states with sponsored dispensaries have their own set of rules and regulations that must be followed in order to adhere to state law.

Once a state has dispensaries, they may be under specific, standardized state rules or the specifics of individual county restrictions on the state law. Again, this varies state by state. Patients should be thoroughly familiar with their state and county laws and regulations regarding their responsibilities and limitations.

Once again, the specifics of how to sign up for a dispensary vary from state to state. In California, where my practice is located, people must attain a certification from their physician, present this with proof of their state residence (usually with a driver's license) to the dispensary, fill out a simple membership form, and allow it to contact the certifying physician to attain permission to dispense medical cannabis. They may register with the state for a fee, but this is not required.

In other states, the specifics will vary. Many states do require registration with the state. This can be an inhibiting factor for those who do not wish for the state to possess this information. While in the state of Washington there are no medical cannabis dispensaries, recreational cannabis shops are allowed to dispense medical cannabis. In most states, the certification to receive medical cannabis is limited to a year, at which time a new certification must be granted. In some other states, the dispensaries are limited to the number and locations the states determine. These dispensaries require state registration with a specific card. In at least one state, the plan is to dispense at specific pharmacies.

The situation is far too diverse and fluid to describe in this book, but other than the states without dispensaries, state laws should be relatively clear about how to join and buy from a dispensary. Unfortunately, this kind of variable picture creates both disparities of available care and opportunity for a continued black market. Despite these problems, diversity of how these laws develop, with an ability to evaluate efficacy and safety with these large-scale and varied models could provide invaluable data for future best practices. This would be unlikely without each state and local community having a substantial part in determining what they will and will not allow.

As states pass recreational cannabis laws, medical dispensary populations are likely to shift. Currently, many people using medical dispensaries are members because of the effects of THC. Most current dispensaries focus on higher-THC products, even when higher-CBD products are available. This is reflective of the low level of knowledge about CBD's benefits as part of an ensemble effect and popular demand for THC containing products.

The myth that cannabis is not effective if the person is not feeling altered is also part of the problem. Even people who enjoy that experience need to be unaltered for most of their day, if they are to be functional members of society. Demand determines supply. As dispensary populations shift, the public is better informed, myths are debunked, and dispensary staffs are better trained, it is likely that medical dispensaries will become the source of high-CBD, THCV, CBDA, CBN, CBG, THCA, CBC, and CBDV strains and embodiments.

DISPLAY OF PRODUCTS

Dispensaries vary in the way they display their products. Some small dispensaries of the farm to medicine cabinet variety or the co-op type do not display the items they have for sale at all. Boutique dispensaries present their items in attractive display cabinets and behind glass walls or cases. The purchaser can examine them to a limited extent in some dispensaries and sample them at others. More elaborate boutique models are evolving in some areas as places people can come and spend time in a relaxed, even elegant atmosphere while trying various products. Some dispensaries are meticulous in their labeling, and deeper TCPs may be available in some dispensaries by request.

Although the latest testing methods are often employed, these phytocannabinoid and terpenoid profiles should be viewed as ballpark figures, rather than as hard and fast numbers. Samples studied may not be from the part of the plant the patient is purchasing, and phytocannabinoid levels can vary from flower to flower.

Additionally, testing is done at a point in time, and the plant's structure keeps changing based on exposure to light, moisture content, temperature, and time. Even tinctures and oils have a volatility that undermines accuracy. However, there is little to be concerned about this, because this shifting phytocannabinoid profile is one reason why the body's disease mechanisms yield to this treatment and have difficulty adapting to and circumventing it.

Still, the figures given about cannabinoid content, while not particularly accurate or stable, are a reasonable starting point to assume what is likely to affect a person in a specific manner. It is always wise, however, to test any new purchase at a time when being altered is safe and unlikely to be critical if psychotropic effects do occur.

Edibles are often attractively displayed and are quite appealing. Again, I would caution that these are the least predictable products, both in consistency and accuracy of labeling. Additionally, they can result in long-term altered states, and should be carefully titrated from far less than recommended doses on the label. Furthermore, they represent an attractive form for children or adults who do not understand that these are cannabis-infused products. If these are to be purchased, they need to be kept in safe and secure areas, beyond prying eyes or uninformed consumption. While movies depicting people who become unintentionally stoned can be hilarious, the reality of this can be quite disconcerting, resulting in many people not wanting to continue treatment or risk to personal safety.

It is especially important to be careful about products labeled to be high in CBD. Often these products are as high or even higher in THC. The idea that a 1:1 edible is not going to cause psychotropic effects is a fallacy, and these effects can be quite long-lasting, especially in the THC-naïve patient. These products are usually best tested in the evening or on a weekend. Additionally, people using edibles need to be willing to be altered, or at least not let that be a deal-breaker. A good time to try edibles is before bedtime, as they can be quite helpful with sustained sleep.

Department store models of dispensaries have massive displays of their products and huge variety. Again, caution with labeling is important. While the variety is impressive, these tend to be the most daunting experiences for novice users. Being an informed consumer is important, but as in all other models of dispensaries, the staff is remarkably helpful and clientele tend to be treated with great respect and dignity. The level of professionalism and breadth of knowledge about cannabis are impressive, but much is subjective, rather than objective science. In general, advice about plant species, strains, and TCPs should be seen as relatively accurate. On the other hand, specific medical conditions' treatments with specific strains or embodiments are often logical but untested. Rather than look at something as treating pain or anxiety, trying different preparations and mixing and matching what is being used to attain best results is the most fruitful way to approach treatment effectiveness. This also emphasizes the importance of variability of the phytocannabinoids for best results and most sculpted and personalized treatment.

ONLINE ORDERING

In many areas, though not in all states, dispensaries have online ordering available. In some areas, online ordering is the only way to order medical cannabis. Legitimate online services for medical cannabis are connected to specific dispensaries. Once a person is accepted as a dispensary member, they can order products online. In general, dedicated delivery services deliver these; however, the US Postal Service is not available for legal transportation of medical cannabis products. Websites vary in quality. Product availability tends to parallel the type of dispensary. Looking at the larger department store model dispensaries, we see the largest inventory and most professional websites.

These are well-tended, highly secure sites, protecting customer identities and using sophisticated software security to prevent cybertheft of accounts. Most of these sites have excellent pictures of their products and reasonably good copy describing items for sale. Some have dedicated educational components to their websites, and some even encourage members to be politically active to advance and protect medical cannabis laws. Boutique sites can also be quite impressive, with a little more homegrown attitude that is really the hallmark of co-operative and farm-to-medicine-cabinet websites. When websites stress high-CBD plants (they are a rarity), they can be the most informative sites about this subject, often with good on-site and linked descriptions, science, current inventory, state-of-the-art information on CBD, and other cannabinoids.

As states legalize recreational cannabis, these websites are likely to shift to reflect their increasing identity as medical sites. In this time of increasing recreational cannabis use, there is likely to be a shakeout between those websites that remain purely medical and those that are either recreational or mixed-use sites. The recreational sites will stress higher THC, and medical sites will initially stress high CBD, then other phytocannabinoids and balanced TCP as the art of medical treatment with cannabis improves over time.

These are evolving ideas, profoundly affected by many local, state, and federal sociocultural issues, evolving law, free-market demands and opportunities, and the shifting sands of political fortunes. One of those sociocultural phenomena is the rise of internet shopping. This trend continues to drive brick-and-mortar stores either into innovating or out of business. Most dispensaries are savvy to the trends on the internet, and will certainly be on the cutting edge of exploiting this sales tool as it becomes more convenient and more dominant.

DELIVERY

Many dispensaries in California use delivery service combined with web ordering to make coming into the dispensary unnecessary. In certain counties in the state, actually going to the dispensary is discouraged, and delivery is the dominant method of dispensing cannabis. For many, this is a good option, because the atmosphere in some dispensaries can be a bit overwhelming. But it is essential to know what one is looking for in a dispensary for online ordering to work, and information for the novice buyer is very confusing. Most places will provide online help or telephone help, but relying on this type of help can be problematic.

There is a lot of information, but it is often inaccurate. The vagaries of medical cannabis labeling and treatment are confusing even for experienced users. The abundance of products; the colorful, stoner-based, uninformative names of products, inaccuracy of labeling content; high-THC product domination; cornucopia of naming conventions; inaccurate, disease-specific treatment labeling; product descriptions focused on experience of the "high"; and lack of web-based orientation for the inexperienced user present a daunting task for many. The sheer convenience of the service offsets this. Online ordering and in-home delivery can be extremely helpful, as well. Otherwise, many extremely ill people would have to go without the option of this treatment in their most debilitated states.

Milieu

The word from most of my patients using medical cannabis is that the people who work in the dispensaries are extremely kind and helpful. This has been a nearly universal experience, and is another factor that separates medical cannabis as a treatment. People in traditional medicine are often caring as well, but there is pressure to get through schedules or to be suspicious of patients abusing their prescriptions that just doesn't exist at the dispensaries. The dispensaries exist to provide access to this care, not to determine whether someone is using that care properly. That is the role of both the patient and their practitioners.

Dispensaries are there to make treatment with medical cannabis available to patients certified by their physicians. As the medical cannabis dispensaries have developed and matured, responsible dispensaries carefully follow state law. They provide the various embodiments of medical cannabis with professional labeling, careful portion control, and clear product information. Budtenders helpfully pass on the knowledge they have from personal experience and from customer feedback.

Standard practices include providing trimmed flowers or buds, tinctures, concentrates, hashish, vaporization oils, strains of clones to grow, topicals, capsules, and edibles. Dispensaries are generally clean and inviting. Some are higher-end and most are designed to be comforting and relaxing.

Having said this, for people being exposed to this treatment for the first time, dispensaries can be intimidating and baffling. Products are impossible to line up with effects from their names. Products with high CBD and low THC sound especially formidable (Cannatonic, Sour Tsunami, etc.). Labels are often inaccurate or inadequate.

Although many dispensaries perform their own testing, these results are really only accurate for the small amount of the plants or embodiments being tested, and will vary from flower to flower, as well as other embodiments, over time. Advice is friendly, but most is THC-oriented, as are the products at the dispensary. Budtenders are very helpful and will often try their best to help patients get products that will not make them high, if they so wish. The problem is that the budtenders know nothing about the patients' sensitivities, and other medical treatments. Furthermore, they have to rely on semi-accurate or inaccurate labeling, as well. Advice may be excellent and well-informed, but how is a customer to know when that is true and when it is not? This is why it is important to start with small quantities and in "protected" time. The sheer volume of product can be overwhelming, as well. Most of my patients want specific, clear recommendations not just about what to use, but how to use it. They need help in following their treatment outcomes, so that they can report progress and it can be reviewed at their appointments. This way, a physician can guide individual treatment through sensible phases, organize an evolving model of improved symptoms and disease management, and distinguish side effects from disease progression or pharmaceutical medical cannabis interactions.

One area of improvement would be in establishing formal mechanisms of communication between the dispensaries and physicians. Since physicians cannot prescribe cannabis, this is different than in pharmacies, where physicians have the sole ability to prescribe. There, they interact with pharmacies by phone, fax, and computer. Dispensaries need liaisons to work with physicians to understand the preferences they have for individual patients. Physicians need to become comfortable with this communication to guide the purchasing decisions of their patients.

Physicians can certainly recommend specific products, but need someone to talk to who is knowledgeable and working specifically in that role at the dispensary. Furthermore, secure communication from the doctor's computer to the dispensary's computer to recommend strains, embodiments, and guidelines for use would be most helpful. Additionally, labeling should be understood as approximate, not precise, even when precise numbers are applied and testing is recent. It would help for dispensaries to separate products by their understood phytocannabinoid profiles, starting with CBD and THC, but expanding to the other known pharmacologically active phytocannabinoids, as well. Doing so would likely determine new treatment paradigms with phytocannabinoid specificity, which could certainly advance treatment. While dispensaries are not pharmacies, they are the hub of treatment procurement, and could become much more than that to benefit their patients, themselves, and treating physicians.

RESEARCH

Dispensaries provide a great place to conduct research. This would include an inventory of products purchased, to determine what the public is purchasing. Furthermore, customer feedback is critical to understanding what is working and not working for patients at dispensaries. Since cannabis is far too complicated and variable a treatment to be studied with normal medical research protocols, collecting data on vast numbers of individuals and analyzing treatment outcomes based on that data is essential. The dispensaries are an excellent place for research and have the huge numbers of patients needed to gather basic information and evaluate it. They can host everything from inventory lists to interviewing individual patients, case series, labeling accuracy, and prospective case series. Protocols need to be developed and tested. This role of the medical cannabis dispensary in research would be invaluable. It would only enhance the credibility of these venues and of the treatment itself.

In conclusion, there are four basic dispensary models, with local variability. Each model has advantages and disadvantages, with the majority taking their role seriously, as provider of genuine medical care with cannabis. Joining a dispensary varies from state to state, but there is usually a clear path to doing so in states that allow dispensaries. Products are often available online for home delivery. The dispensaries themselves are easily accessible with the correct medical certification. They tend to be clean, efficient, and well organized. While product content is prominently displayed, it is often inaccurate. This is not an attempt to subvert the truth, but is most often related to the changing nature of the plant before, during, and after harvest, as well as in any and all embodiments. Dispensaries need to go beyond the current high-THC dominance to balanced CBD:THC, high-CBD, and raw plant preparations.

Furthermore, dispensaries and growers need to be more concerned about evaluating the larger TCP of individual strains, so that treatment options can be more precisely directed, while broadening clinical effectiveness of treatment. Both dispensaries and physicians need to develop ways to communicate with each other to improve care. Furthermore, dispensaries provide an ideal opportunity to collect big data, so necessary to establish directions of care and to help refine and develop the science of medical cannabis treatment.

Chapter 6

Paraphernalia

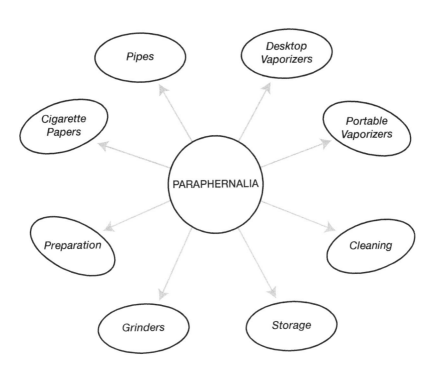

Getting started with medical cannabis treatment can be confusing enough. Collecting and incorporating the paraphernalia to help this happen is another important area to be understood and applied. The states have different laws about paraphernalia available for cannabis, which must be evaluated before purchasing or possessing it. In a state such as Florida, only use of high-CBD, extremely low THC tincture is allowed, while possession of paraphernalia for cannabis use is illegal.

The traditional way to consume cannabis is in a hand-rolled cigarette or with different types of pipes. Now, there are various ways of vaporizing it instead of smoking it. Although there are no proven benefits of vaporizing over smoking, it does remove most of the tars from the experience. It makes sense to limit the health risks as much as possible. Vaporizers are varied in portability, convenience, efficiency, vaporization method, cannabis embodiment, and many other factors. Although the flowers can be ground with one's hands, a grinder is the preferred method. However, grinding for loading in a pipe or vaporizing is quite different from making capsules. Tools for putting cannabis in capsule form also vary from plastic pen covers to chromed instruments or capsule makers. Storage of cannabis and its preparations is yet another important consideration. Accessories from screen-cleaning products to water cooling are available in a myriad of choices. Additionally, storage of cannabis and accessories plays another role in preserving and transforming the raw plant into something medically useful. Capsule-making and other preparation equipment are helpful to understand how to make the medical cannabis patient's experience more organized and pleasurable. In this chapter, I will look at many of these choices to help clarify the multiple options available to prepare various embodiments for consumption, while keeping the plant fresh and retaining potency.

Different people not only seek out different experience of the effects of medical cannabis, they also consume it in different ways. Chapter 4 emphasizes development of treatment in three phases, beginning (tolerability, some symptom relief), intermediate (increased TCP) profound symptom relief and advanced (rotating TCP) restoration of balance and health. The idea is to develop a broad TCP and a varied treatment approach. Early treatment should be aimed at tolerability and symptom control, moving through later phases of deeper symptom relief and restoration of normal health and balance. Having said this, everyone pursuing this treatment will come up with their own routines of use. This is preferable to regimented directions. What works well for one person will make another person too uncomfortable.

The paraphernalia used for consumption is just as personal a decision at one level, but using this treatment in various forms provides a differentiation of treatment from rapid onset of symptom relief to deep and long-lasting control of illness and health. Cannabis is something people have used for millennia. It can be prepared for consumption without any device, but good preparation greatly aids variability of use. This can be as simple as rolling cigarette papers or a pipe and lighter to $600 or more for a tabletop vaporizer or elaborate water pipe. Some people will be happiest with the largest collection of the highest-quality tools. Others will want to keep things as basic and simple as possible. There are no rules. Instead, there are only a broad array of choices to customize the experience to fit one's personality and lifestyle. Remembering that one of the endocannabinoid system's main functions is to maintain pleasure and wellbeing, using medical cannabis to enhance and work on that enhanced system should be a happy experience.

No discussion of medical cannabis paraphernalia could start anywhere other than cigarette-rolling papers. These remain the simplest, most common way to consume the plant. Rolling ground or crushed cannabis into a marijuana cigarette "joint" is accomplished by placing the flowers and leaves in a rolling paper, rolling it up, licking the glued side, lighting it, and inhaling.

The advantage of this approach is its simplicity. This is relatively easy to learn. Rolling a joint has been a rite of passage for those using cannabis recreationally for decades. For medical cannabis, the joint is still the most popular form of cannabis consumption, but many use vaporizers instead. Although smoking cannabis in a joint is simple, there are more convenient methods of consumption. Edibles, tinctures, capsules, cannabis oil, and even vapor from a portable vaporizer can all be consumed more quickly and more privately. Since using medical cannabis requires a certain etiquette of not forcing oneself on others, ways other than smoking a joint to pursue this treatment become essential.

Questions about the safety of smoked or inhaled cannabis became a raging subject after publication of a paper stating that there were three times more tars in cannabis than tobacco. This led to the erroneous conclusions that cannabis was likely to cause lung cancer and that the rate was likely to be worse than with cigarettes. In a subsequent study done on lung cancer victims in the greater Los Angeles area by the same author, it turned out that not only was cannabis less likely to cause lung cancer than cigarettes, but that regular cannabis smokers had lower lung cancer rate than cigarette smokers and non-smokers. Several other studies have confirmed this result.[126,127]

The problem with this type of analysis, however is that it is similar to asking if food causes cancer or if pharmaceuticals are risks for heart damage. Some foods and drugs are higher-risk, some are lower-risk, and some may reduce the risk. Cannabis is not one substance or one type of treatment. It is as infinite as food choices and preparations, so no generalizations can be made about the plant or its users. Smoked cannabis varies in its anti-tumor effects because it varies in TCP from one strain to another. This has a significant and varied effect on the body. One thing everybody knows is that

---

126   Huang Y-HJ et al. An epidemiologic review of marijuana and cancer: an update. *Cancer Epidemiology Biomarkers & Prevention* 24, no. 1 (2014): 15–31.

127   Tashkin DP. Effects of marijuana smoking on the lung. *Annals of the American Thoracic Society* (2013): 10, no. 3, 239–247.

cannabis makes the user high . . . except there are now many strains that are available that do not, and they tend to fetch a higher price than those that do. Additionally, there are several ways to use strains that will make the user high if smoked that do not in other forms or uses, such as raw or topical.

That said, most users will smoke marijuana, most of the time. Considering the massive and long-term use of cannabis in the smoked form, where is the worldwide public health crisis caused by this practice? The answer is that, to date, with millions of person-years of use (people who have smoked cannabis times the number of years they have done so), it does not exist. In fact, looking at large population retrospective and prospective open studies shows the exact opposite, with cannabis exhibiting efficacy in reduction of deaths in post-traumatic brain injury,[128] brain hemorrhage-related illness,[129] opioid withdrawal,[130] cancer symptom severity,[131] Crohn's disease severity.[132] The only thing that could even begin to be construed as a public health problem related to cannabis use is the social and financial costs of incarcerating so many young recreational users. The cost of this to our society is immense, a terrible consequence of a wrongheaded drug policy that needs immediate correction and reconciliation.

One of the problems with smoking cannabis is the distinctive smell, and the risk that this smell carries with it if law enforcement discovers the user. That said, it is still likely that the least healthy

---

128   Nguyen BM et al. Effects of marijuana use on outcomes of Traumatic Brain Injury. *American Journal of Surgery* 80, no. 10 (2014): 979–983.

129   Di Napoli M et al. Prior Cannabinoid use is associated with outcomes after intracerebral hemorrhage. *Cerebrovascular Disease* 41, no. 5 (2016): 248–255.

130   Scavone JL et al. Impact of cannabis use during stabilization on methadone maintenance. *American Journal of Addiction* 22, no. 4 (2013): 344–351.

131   Waisengrin B et al. Patters of use of medical cannabis among Israeli cancer patients: a single institution experience. *Journal of Pain and Symptom Management* 49, no. 2 (2015): 223–230.

132   Naftali T et al. Treatment of Crohn's disease with cannabis: a naturalistic study. *Israeli Medical Association Journal* 13, no. 8 (2011): 455–458.

way to consume marijuana is smoking it. There are more tars in marijuana than tobacco, but there is no nicotine. The amount of cannabis consumed certainly pales to the amount of tobacco used by its users. This may be part of the reason there is so little significant lung disease of any sort among users. The other reason, however, is that at the base of most chronic illness is local and cell-specific inflammation. Tobacco is both highly inflammatory, due to tars, and highly addictive, due to nicotine. Cannabis is highly anti-inflammatory. It achieves this with multiple phytocannabinoids blocking multiple inflammatory cascades, while mounting multiple anti-inflammatory resolutions. This means that many of the negative effects of smoking cannabis are countered by the positive health benefits of the actual phytocannabinoids, especially since at least seven of them are anti-inflammatory. The public belief that this relates to THC and CBD is only partially correct. Below is a table showing some of the benefits of the plant-based phytocannabinoids.

TABLE 14: MAJOR PHYTOCANNABINOID HEALTH BENEFITS

	THC	CBD	THCA	CBDA	CBC	CBN	THCV
Analgesia	Yes	Yes	Yes	Yes	Yes	Yes	
Anit-Inflammatory	Yes	Yes	Yes	Yes	Yes	Yes	
Anti-Cancer	Yes	Yes	Yes	Yes	Yes	Yes	
Anti-Anxiety	Yes	Yes					
Anti-Epilepsy	Yes	Yes					Yes
Anti-Nausea	Yes	Yes	Yes	Yes			
Neuroprotective	Yes	Yes	Yes				
Metabolic Syndrome		Yes		Yes			Yes
Well Being	Yes	Yes	Yes				

Even the above table is too simplified, because it is not merely the effects of the various phytocannabinoids that are important. It is the way that they interact with each other and the endocannabinoid system that makes this treatment approach so remarkable. This synergy of the plant phytocannabinoids, how they interact with the body's endocannabinoid (pleasure, wellbeing, energy, and balance) system, plus the positive interaction of both of these systems with the endorphin system (pain relief and regulation of the continuum between pleasure and pain), vanilloid system (temperature regulation, conversion of chronic pain to acute pain, bone formation and breakdown), PPAR-Gamma system (blood sugar regulation, weight gain and weight loss, serum lipid levels, new nerve cell formation), catecholamine system (mood, reward, sleep, and energy), GABA/glutamate system (nerve cell inhibition and excitation, anxiety, and pleasure), hormonal system (myriad body regulatory and modifying substances), and immune system (acute inflammation and chronic inflammation) creates an astonishing number of opportunities to restore balance and wellbeing.

The big advantages of smoking the plant are the rapidity of onset of its activity and the extremely high but relatively short-lived blood levels of multiple cannabinoids. In medicine, inhaled substances tend to have very rapid onsets. Cannabis is no exception, with peak blood levels being attained within 90 seconds to 5 minutes. Blood levels 20 to 50 times higher than edible levels are quickly attained and eliminated within 15 minutes. Tissue activity lasts for 2–3 hours. Compared to treatment with orally consumed cannabis, which achieve high tissue levels due to low but long-lasting blood levels, inhaled cannabis is rapidly in and out of the system, while oral cannabis is slow in onset, but much longer-lasting.

There may be psychological addiction issues with either inhaled or oral cannabis, but physiologic addiction is nonexistent. Because the psychoactive components of cannabinoids activate dopamine-based reward circuits, and because the endocannabinoid system regulates pleasure, there is certainly a drive to consume psychoactive forms of the plant. People who do so can routinely step away from it, however, without suffering any physiologic withdrawal. This same reward system works with medical cannabis. The long-term feeling of wellbeing with this treatment leads to a high retention rate among users. Because this treatment is not suppressive of other systems and promotes positive neuroplastic change as well as pleasurable experience, the brain's pleasure, reward, and salience chemistry reinforces use. This does not require feeling high. Instead, it is focused on a sense of wellness and wellbeing.

Other than a marijuana cigarette, cannabis can be inhaled in various pipes. These may be portable and fairly stealthy forms or elaborate, large desktop glass-sculpted water pipes that are genuine works of art. The water can serve to cool the cannabis, presenting a less inflammatory substance to the upper and lower respiratory tracts. There are even pipes that can be refrigerated with smoke pathways that pass through a cooled column of glycerin, further cooling the smoke.

Vaporizers are even more remarkable because they remove a lot of the tars by not burning the plants to activate THCA to THC and CBDA to CBD. Instead they heat the plant only enough to remove the water vapor that performs the transformation, but leaves most of the tars behind. Vaporizers can be large desktop models, such as the best-known, Volcano. These sometimes fill balloons with vapor, and then the user inhales the content of the balloons. This approach not only lowers consumption of tars, but also cools the vapor. These can also be used with inhalation of the vapor directly from the heat source. Many medical users find the balloon method to be too elaborate, however, and prefer a simpler approach.

Perhaps the best vaporizer embodiment of all is the portable vaporizer. It needs no external heat source, produces clean vapor, and is very easy to carry around. Vaporizers most often have digital displays that range from multiple predetermined settings to degree-by-degree adjustments. These vaporizers are generally designed for short-term use between charges, but may also use interchangeable batteries or quick charge modes. Some models also may be used while being charged. Portable vaporizers can be large enough to stretch the boundaries of the "portable" category or can be easily carried in the pocket.

Vaporizers can be used to vaporize concentrated cannabis oil, plant material, or concentrated cannabis solids. These solids are also known as "shatter," "wax," "waxy oils," "butter" or "hash oil." These differences have more to do with the consistency of the preparation than differences in potency. Cannabis oil and shatter tend to be highly concentrated and are usually extremely high in THC. Occasionally they are low in THC and very high in CBD, but these are much harder to find, especially in shatter. Shatter is best for only experienced users, while vaporizable cannabis oils are a more reliable concentrate. Still, these concentrates are much higher in cannabinoids than the plant flowers or tinctures, so they need to be consumed with moderation and care. Vaporizing cannabis oil can be very convenient and emits almost no telltale scent. Some concentrates come in capsules or in syringes, but doses are not reliable. These are consumed orally and can lead to long-lasting and frightening side effects, such as vomiting, panic, and paranoia. It cannot be emphasized enough that before medical cannabis users try even high-CBD concentrates, they should start low, during non-obligated, safe time, and be prepared to have a much more intense high and perhaps have to sleep off effects.

Both edibles and concentrates are most responsible for ER visits among people using cannabis recreationally and some medical users as well. Having said this, they can be more economical and deliver doses needed for treating medical problems, especially when very high CBD levels are desirable. One of the problems with highly concentrated THC doses is that they can cross from being anti-inflammatory, anti-anxiety, and anti-nausea to pro-inflammatory, anxiety-producing, and nausea-promoting. An alternative to concentrates is to mix use of tinctures with vaporized flowers and preheated and unheated cannabis bud capsules. In this manner, the broadest cannabis profiles are delivered. There is also concern about the residual aspects of even purged concentrates, which can retain solvent or metabolic products of the solvents used to concentrate them, even after purging. Additionally, while cannabinoids are concentrated, so are contaminants, such as residual solvent and pesticides. Testing once the product is delivered to the dispensary is of extra importance, regarding health and wellbeing. Do not trust manufacturer certification, as it may not accurately reflect individual batches prepared with this method.

Advantages to concentrates include removal of more tar producing plant material. There has never been any evidence that there is any health benefit between vaporizing plant material or vaporizing oil, but this lack of medical evidence is not unusual for cannabis consumption in general. That there are little or no residual tars left behind from vaporizing cannabis oil points to the relative decrease in tars in cannabis oil, compared to the flowers of the plant. It also removes many of the terpenes found in the plant. Even non-cannabinoid terpenes add anti-inflammatory, anti-microbial properties to medical cannabis treatment, however. So, removing them may create a decrease in the plant's overall synergistic medical effects.

One of the issues with vaporizers is that they tend to work best with a coarse grind, but not too coarse. Grinders are mechanical devices that accept the dried bud of cannabis flowers. They grind the buds to a degree of coarseness determined by their design and the user's desire. Grinders come in two, three, and four stages, although it is easiest to get two or four stages currently.

A two-stage grinder has teeth in its upper and lower parts, held closed by a magnet. Ground cannabis sinks to the bottom of the grinder and needs to be dumped onto another surface to load cigarette, pipe, or vaporizer. How much material there is determines the degree of the grind. These grinders usually are made of aluminum, but there are wooden ones available. The back-and-forth motion of the grinder adds a pleasant tactile experience to grinding medical cannabis, and after initial resistance to the process, grinders are smooth to use. Tactile and auditory feedback are good predictors of when the grind is complete. Two-stage grinders give the finest grind.

Three- and four-stage grinders have specifically sized holes in the bottom of the grind chamber, to let the grind come through and into an accessible bottom chamber. In four-stage chambers, a shallow screened chamber is screwed into the bottom grinder collector, allowing pollen to be collected below. The results can be scraped up and added to joint, pipe, or vaporizer. They can also be collected and placed into a pollen press, where two screw-down tops and inserts pressurize the pollen to make a block of it known as kief. If a low heat source is added to the press (metal parts only), the kief will rupture the pollen further, and the resin will result in hashish, the original cannabis concentrate. While inexpensive grinders can be quite effective, the higher the quality of the grinding teeth, the less likely it is that any metal shavings will get in the ground cannabis. Grinders also come in the form of cards for simple grinding onto paper, tabletops, or trays. They come in various sizes, but small ones are best for portability. Medium and large grinders are best for home use. If a person can only have one grinder, a medium-sized, four-staged grinder is probably the best choice. Portability is compromised, but this can always be managed by pre-grinding and carrying the ground plant in an odor-concealing storage container.

Another way to consume cannabis is in capsules. This is best done with a very fine grind available with an electric coffee grinder. Capsules can be made from preheated cannabis or the raw plant. Each has its own advantages, and the real magic occurs in combining them.

Combinations can be done using separate capsules or within one capsule, as preferred. Keeping them in separate capsules makes them easier to catalogue, so use of a particular strain will be known. Preheating higher-THCA plants will activate THCA to THC, but the body's metabolic processing will not. The same is true for other acidic forms of the plant, but the body will transform CBDA to CBD. As stated earlier, this happens even more efficiently than heating the plant. In medical treatment, using raw capsules of a high-CBDA plant will provide blood and tissue levels of CBD and CBDA. If one wishes to avoid the psychotropic effects of cannabis, a preheated, high-CBDA, low-THCA capsule or a raw capsule of any combination of phytocannabinoids should do the trick. The broadest phytocannabinoid blood and tissue levels will combine both approaches.

Some people will become altered with raw high THCA, and must test this approach in a safe and protected time. For sleep or to have the effect of a high-THC edible experience, a high-THCA plant preheated then ground and placed in a capsule is usually effective. Again, caution is advised for novice users. Cannabis naive or not, capsules should always be tested during times when being altered is acceptable. Empty capsules are available in most vitamin shops, health food stores or online. Look for vegetarian capsules that range from small #3 capsules up to large #00 capsules. Starting small and pure is best to determine if there are any psychotropic effects with any particular strain. Although advanced users will want to combine various strains or combine cannabis with other herbal treatments, it is always best to start with pure capsules. The capsules themselves have a large and small side. It is advisable to fill the small side first, then cap and lock with the large side to determine tolerability. Once this is clear, switching to filling the large side first is an excellent approach. These capsule halves can be locked down on each other by placing the ends between the thumb and forefinger, then squeezing until feeling a noticeable clunk. It is usually not necessary to start with a #3 capsule, as these are quite small. A good starting off place is a #1 capsule, but these are a bit harder to find than #0 or #00. The large capsules can be used to start treatment with less cannabis used to fill them. Even in the capsule form, light, air, humidity, temperature, and time will all create a changing phytocannabinoid profile. Storing capsules in a dark, cool place will be more likely to preserve a TCP closest to the original profile of the plant when harvested. This is nothing to get too concerned about, remembering that part of this treatment at its most sophisticated is to create a rotating or constantly changing TCP.

This ushers in the important topic of cannabis storage. The ideal storage environment for cannabis in dried flower form is in jars open to the air at 62% humidity in a humidor. The typical cigar humidor is kept at 70–75%, but this is too moist for storage of cannabis. Boveda makes packets that regulate humidity inside of humidors or other storage containers by exchanging humidity with the surrounding air. It makes these for the storage of many products, and is a leading vendor for use in cigar humidors. For these, it provides a 72% packet, too high in humidity for cannabis. It has also made a 62% packet for use with medical cannabis, in several sizes to accommodate different sized storage containers. The result is the ability to taper the size or number of packets to fit the size of the storage container and the weight of the stored cannabis.

While cigar humidors are fine for storing cannabis, they will impart the flavor of Spanish cedar used to line their inside compartments to the cannabis. For some, this is not acceptable, but it does nothing to degrade the plant phytocannabinoid and terpenoid profiles. Many cannot taste the change in cannabis flavor and cigar humidors can work well for long term storage. If using a Boveda62 packet, it is best to not use another form of humidity control, such as those included with humidors, as each method will fight the other and make for less reliable control of internal humidity. Cannador makes humidors for cannabis that do not use Spanish cedar. Instead, they use more neutral wood, such as mahogany. They also have storage containers made of glass, with plastic tops that let varying amounts of air into the container to exchange humidity with the environment.

Cannabis should be stored in containers, not just placed in the humidor directly. Additionally, the traditional plastic baggy is not a good way to store cannabis, and should not be used other than for transport. Makeshift containers can be found in kitchen stores that open to the air in varying fashion, and can be closed off completely if desired. An option to containers stored in humidors is the C-Vault, an opaque stainless-steel container that has a slot for the appropriately sized Boveda62 packet. Both the Boveda62 and the C-Vault come in multiple sizes adapted to each other. Storing in clear glass canning jars and mason jars is fine, but these should be kept in a cool dark place with an appropriately sized Boveda62 packet stored with the cannabis inside the jar.

Prep trays are used as spillovers. One may already own a tray that can serve in this way, or one may buy a specialty tray made for preparing and cleaning up after grinding the plant. One can chop the plant on top of the tray by hand or with a knife. One can also dump the contents of a two-staged grinder or flat grinder onto it. Specialty trays come with a card, and one corner is sometimes open for easy cleanup and to sweep the residual cannabis back into its appropriate container. This can be important when cleaning various strains of cannabis on the same tray, so not to inadvertently mix high-potency THC cannabis with low, preventing unwanted psychotropic effects.

Cleaning products for vaporizers and pipes include pipe cleaners, swabs, rubbing alcohol, and special cleaning fluids. Rubbing alcohol and pipe cleaners are ideal and effective for cleaning screens, vapor path, and bowls. While other commercial products are available, they are not more effective than these two, and in this case, simpler is better. If a deep cleaning is needed, immersing screens in the alcohol is effective. These should be allowed to cool before doing so. This can be followed with the use of a pipe cleaner. Alcohol should be allowed to evaporate before adding a heat source. The inside of a cooled vaporizer bowl can usually be cleaned with alcohol on a pipe cleaner or swab, but follow manufacturer instructions to be sure. Pipe bowls can be cleaned with alcohol and pipe cleaner or swab, while screens can be soaked in alcohol. Again, remember to allow the alcohol to evaporate off before applying a heat source.

TABLE 15: MEDICAL CANNABIS PARAPHERNALIA

Paraphernalia	Preparation	Consumption
Desktop Vaporizers	Plug into wall or use wirelessly if this feature is available. Use with a balloon or separately with an inhalation tube supplied with the vaporizer. Balloon provides cooler inhalation, Grind up medical cannabis coarsest between the fingers or with a grinder. Not portable.	Generate vapor with either method. Slow deep inhalation. Even without visible vapor, phytocannabinoids are delivered in a rapid fashion. Less tars than smoked. Usually deliver large clouds of vapor. LED or digital displays let user know when proper temperature is reached.
Portable Vaporizers	Rechargeable batteries. Portability varies from large and heavier models to those that are light and easily carried. Heavier models tend to have better battery life, but portable models can be quite long lasting. Grind up medical cannabis coarsest between the fingers or finest with a grinder.	Vapor is generated by inhaling near or distant from heating chamber. Conduction and convection heating are each used, but convection less likely to burn cannabis. Less tars than smoked. Usually deliver smaller vapor clouds. LED or digital displays let user know when proper temperature is reached.

Paraphernalia	Preparation	Consumption
Grinder	Metal and wood grinders are both available. Quality varies tremendously. They all get the job done, but metal grinders made of machined aircraft grade aluminum are best and wood grinders with metal teeth are also an excellent choice.	Medical Cannabis Flowers are placed in the grinder. Come in two, three and four stage forms. Four stage grinders collect pollen through a screened chamber and have a collecting chamber for storage of ground flower. Two stage grinder allows for finer grind. Grind back and forth for finer grind or grind in constant direction for faster grind.
Other Accessories	Prep trays, pollen presses, cleaning products, humidors, cases, storage containers	Specific functions vary regarding purpose of product. Prep trays- trays to prepare consumables. Pollen press- makes compressed Kief or Hashish to smoke or vaporize. Cleaning products- clean pipes, screens, vaporizers. Humidor- store plant at 62% humidity. Cases- store and transport paraphernalia. Storage containers- safely store plant products

Accessories play an important role in using medical cannabis. Use can be managed without this paraphernalia, but such devices help make the experience easier and more pleasurable. This chapter reviewed many of the types of products available, but certainly does not cover them all. All of this is available for online ordering, and usually discreetly packaged. Because of the illegality of cannabis at the federal level in the United States, the companies that make these products are careful to make disclaimers and refer to "herbal substances" rather than cannabis. The creativity and professional quality of these products is quite high and comprises a large industry, albeit an industry that would be much more limited without states enacting medical cannabis laws. The next chapter will deal with the quasi-legal status of this treatment option and look at the current state of the law and medical cannabis use, sale, and distribution in the United States. It would be impossible to cover the rest of the world, but this information is usually available on the internet. This is an area in considerable flux, and should not be confused with recreational cannabis laws enacted by several states. If planning to use medical cannabis, check state regulations before doing so to make sure that the use of this treatment does not violate state and local ordinances. Currently, forty-four states and the District of Columbia that have passed laws for use of medical cannabis, but many of these are not yet finalized or activated, and they are widely varied in what is legal and what is not.

Chapter 7

We Fought the Law
... And We Won

THE HISTORY OF STATES APPROVING medical cannabis as a treatment started with California, and built steam throughout most of the United States over the next twenty years. In many states, the law is recent enough to become the law but not yet be implemented. It all started with Proposition 215 passing in California in 1996. Since then, the pattern has been one of activism and public pressure to legalize medical cannabis, followed by states coming up with actual legislation to make this treatment available. Different states have restricted use to specific serious conditions, with some states opening it up to physicians' discretion, but most controlled by legislative or executive action. The law has lagged behind the will of the people, creating confusion and vacuum. This in turn has led to an expansion and contraction of regulations, aimed initially at limiting use and more recently at revenue generation.

Another problem is that of law enforcement. Law enforcement is in as much flux as the actual treatment with medical cannabis. Law officers are used to the war on drugs, and #1 on that list for arrests and incarcerations is marijuana. State laws have shifted, but old habits die hard. Moving from strict enforcement of a serious drug crime to dealing with appropriate medical use can be quite unsettling for people in law enforcement. There is a general cynicism about marijuana as a medical treatment, and this is not unique to law enforcement.

All this hinders smooth transitions, but despite this, medical cannabis as a treatment continues to gain momentum. The best current updates of state laws and local legal issues can be found on norml.org. The longest experience remains in the state of California, which is transitioning from a law guaranteeing access to a law designed to bring the current, quasi-legal, cash-based business model to one of helping businesses pay state and federal taxes to maintain a vibrant economic model, while bringing in revenues to the state. California is also trying to transition from a specialized set of physicians making yearly certifications for this treatment to treating physicians treating their patients and following them after certification to give advice and make changes in treatment planning, as if cannabis were any other treatment. This is an attempt to reel in the treatment, but also to make it more medically mainstream. The federal government has passed laws to give states with medical cannabis laws room to see how this works out, but still restricts banks from providing accounts to cannabis businesses, seriously limiting the ability for these programs to operate "above ground." There is a struggle between state and federal rights to determine this policy, with both sides trying to figure out ways to cooperate with each other around the issue of self-determinism for states.

Looming over this is the failed war on drugs, with its many constructs that make it hard for the federal government to find a way to support this treatment beyond a basic "don't ask, don't tell" policy. After decades of incarcerating offenders for possession and selling of cannabis, local law enforcement has no trust in this treatment and faces considerable problems regulating it in the context of existing laws. The DEA has continued to make all plant-based cannabis products, including the non-psychoactive CBD, Schedule-1, illegal with no medicinal value. This probably saved a lot of chaos by not foisting total and sole prescribing of this treatment to physicians, who are currently not properly educated to carry this out. Making cannabis or its components a Schedule-2 drug would have made them illegal to acquire without a special prescription. Physicians can make recommendations, but are currently unable to write prescriptions. This has resulted in an uncomfortable truce between patients and their government. To its credit, Congress has tried to create a structure of change that has received bipartisan support, but this still needs to be permanently worked out. Everyone appears to be waiting for medical science to catch up to the public will, but this is unlikely to be a satisfactory solution. Medical science is way behind the knowledge curve on the subject. It will take some time to catch up, if it ever does. The medicinal value of the plant is established beyond any shadow of doubt, but the ability to use current standards of medical evidence to verify this is completely inadequate. To date, only one medical school, the University of Colorado, has included medical cannabis in its curriculum. The tragedy here is that the endocannabinoid system continues to be the victim of collateral damage, buried in obscurity. It is a critical disease modifying system and begs to be moved to the forefront of medical education and treatment.

Big Pharma is pushing for drugs that will replace cannabis at the cost of safety, while ignoring the safety record of the plant. That safety record is so impressive that it should be the gold standard to measure the safety of pharmaceuticals. However, organized medicine has historically been more comfortable with standard single drug formulations than with plant-based medicines. This is also more comfortable for the general public, which prefers mass-produced, safe, standardized products to herbal treatments. While Big Pharma is unpopular these days, the lifesaving treatments it has developed are legion. It will continue to be involved in developing and using cannabinoids to treat illness.

Companies in other countries such as Israel are trying to find ways to help patients, physicians, and Big Pharma. These companies have come up with effective products and delivery systems for this treatment. Once the United States joins in more actively, the progress of these approaches will pick up and become more profitable. The patient will then benefit.

But today, cannabis remains an illegal drug with big prison terms potentially there for all involved. It is time for the plant to be freed up from the entire scheduling of drugs. At this point, many states have allowed legal cultivation, and huge cannabis-growing operations already exist. Scheduling something grown by the metric ton is highly questionable to begin with, but denying the public access to the plant's medical benefits makes absolutely no sense at all.

Adoption of cannabis will certainly disrupt existing laws, calling for a reconciliation. There are obvious problems, such as driving while impaired or operating complex equipment under the influence, but less obvious problems also exist, such as the severe mental impairment experienced by some users. This is no different than use of current prescribed medication and resulting impairment conflicts with current law.

Decriminalization, with penalties for breaking existing non-drug-related laws under the influence, needs to be instituted nationwide. As with alcohol, prohibition has led to organized crime stepping into the breach. It has also criminalized millions of people, who would not consider anything of a criminal nature under other circumstances. This undermines the authority of law enforcement and the rule of law. Tragically, lives have been lost and destroyed for use of a plant that can be employed to reduce anxiety, post-traumatic stress disorder, aggression, depression, and fear. We don't jail people for using turmeric or lavender medicinally, but millions have been jailed and worse for using cannabis, and millions are in jail still.

In the checkerboard of state laws regarding medical cannabis, a slowly evolving change is inexorable. 1930s politics are yielding to the national conscience of the 21st century. The public will has created a demand that allows state and local governments to challenge the status quo, without trying to keep afloat in a raging sea of ignorance. Lawmakers are often fearful of introducing a change that goes against publicly held beliefs. Remember, only a short while ago, interracial marriage was illegal in several states. It took a constitutional amendment to give women the right to vote.

This is certainly an opportunity for state and federal government to raise funds without a general tax increase for a group of people who would gladly trade higher taxation on cannabis for fully legal access. While allowing each state to determine its own laws addresses its own needs, there will need to be a better overarching federal structure to medical and recreational cannabis that will allow the free market to develop, but will provide cohesive guidelines and sharing of state and federal taxes on cannabis.

The following table delineates U.S. states and territories' medical cannabis laws, evaluated by NORML as of January of 2017:

Table 16: State by State Medical Cannabis Law

State	Type of Law	Conditions	Patient Possession Limit	Home Cultivation	Dispensaries	Caregivers
AL	CBD	Epilepsy	Unclear	No	No	No
AK	CBD	Epilepsy	Unclear	No	No	No
AZ	Medical	Multiple	2.5 oz	12 if 25 miles from dispensary	Yes	Yes
AR	Medical (not yet operational)	Multiple	No limit specified	No	Yes	No
CA	Medical	Multiple and physician discretion	No limit specified	Yes No limit specified	Yes	Yes
CO	Medical	Multiple	2 oz	6 plants (3 mature)	Yes	Yes
CT	Medical	Multiple	1 month's worth	No	Yes	Yes
DE	Medical	Multiple	6 oz	No	Yes	No
DC	Medical	Physician Discretion	2 oz	No	Yes	Yes
FL	CBD	Multiple	Unclear	No	Yes-home delivery	No
GA	THC<5% CBD > or = to THC	Multiple	20 oz of infused cannabis oil	No	No	No
HI	Medical	Multiple	4 oz	13 plants	Yes	Yes
IL	Medical	Multiple	2.5 oz every 14 days	No	Yes, but not operational	Yes

State	Type of Law	Conditions	Patient Possession Limit	Home Cultivation	Dispensaries	Caregivers
IA	CBD	Intractable Epilepsy	"Limited amounts of CBD oil"	No	No	No
KY	CBD	Intractable Epilepsy	Unclear	No	No	No
LA	Medical (Not Operational)	Multiple	30 days of non-smokable	No	10 Pharmacies	No
MA	Medical	Physician Determined	10 oz every 2 months	Yes (unclear amounts)	Yes	Yes
MD	Medical (Not operational)	Multiple	30 days	No	Yes	No
ME	Medical	Multiple	2.5 oz	6 mature plants	Yes	Yes
MI	Medical	Multiple	2.5 oz	12 plants	Yes	Yes
MN	Medical	Multiple	30 days non-smokable	No	Yes	No
MS	CBD	Intractable Epilepsy	Extracts with at least 15% CBD <0.5% THC	No	No	No
MO	CBD	Intractable Epilepsy	20 oz Extracts with >5% CBD and < 0.3% THC	No	Yes (Not Operational)	No
MT	Medical	Multiple	1 oz	4 plants plus 12 seedlings	Yes	Yes

State	Type of Law	Conditions	Patient Possession Limit	Home Cultivation	Dispensaries	Caregivers
NV	Medical	Multiple	2.5 oz	12 plants	Yes	Yes
NH	Medical	Multiple	2 oz	No	Yes	No
NJ	Medical	Multiple	2 oz per month	No	Yes	Yes
NM	Medical	Multiple	8oz per 90 days	16 plants (4 mature)	Yes	Yes
NY	Medical	Multiple	30 days non-smokable	No	Yes	Yes
NC	CBD	Intractable Epilepsy	Extracts with <0.9% THC and >5% CBD	No	No	No
ND	Medical (Not operational)	Multiple	Up to 4 oz	12 plants if >40 miles from a dispensary	Yes	Unknown
OH	Medical (Not operational)	Multiple	Oils, tinctures, extracts, edibles, patches, herbal material	No	Yes	No
OK	CBD	Pediatric Epilepsy	<0.3% THC from stems and seeds only	No	No	No
OR	Medical	Multiple	24 oz	6 mature plants, 18 seedlings	Yes	Yes
PA	Medical (Not operational)	Multiple	oil, tinctures, topicals, liquid	No	Yes	Yes

State	Type of Law	Conditions	Patient Possession Limit	Home Cultivation	Dispensaries	Caregivers
PR	Medical	Multiple	30 day supply non-smokable	No	Yes	No
RI	Medical	Multiple	2.5 oz	12 plants and 12 seedlings	Yes	Yes
SC	CBD	epilepsy	Extracts >15% CBD and < 0.9% THC	No	No	No
TN	CBD	Intractable seizures	Extracts <0.9% THC	No	No	No
TX	CBD (non-functional)	epilepsy	THC < 5% CBD > 10%	No	No	No
UT	CBD	Intractable epilepsy	extracts with >15% CBD and <0.3% THC	No	No	No
VT	Medical	Multiple	2 oz	9 total plants- 2 mature	Yes	Yes
VA	CBD	Intractable Epilepsy	Extracts >15%CBD <5% THC	No	No	No
WA	Medical	Physician determined	3 oz of plant 48 oz of solid 21 grams of concentrates 216 ounces of liquids	6 plants with up to 8 oz of usable cannabis	No, but retailers for recreational cannabis can supply medical cannabis	Yes

State	Type of Law	Conditions	Patient Possession Limit	Home Cultivation	Dispensaries	Caregivers
WI	CBD	epilepsy	CBD without psychotropic effect	No	No	No
WY	CBD	intractable epilepsy	CBD extract <0.3% THC from Hemp	No	No	No

This is quite a list of states and territories that have legalized cannabis in some form, despite the position of the federal government. These individual states and often their direct voting populations, came up with new laws to extend the use of cannabis for compassionate medical treatment. Some states are highly restrictive about this use, but still, only six states in the country do not have some compassionate use law. Most medical cannabis laws are on the books because the people wanted this treatment. This is a potential revenue generator for the states, but more importantly, it presents unique medical opportunities to advance the treatment of many difficult conditions as well as more easily treated ones. The states have charged ahead of the federal government, which has shown the wisdom to allow the states to figure out their own rules, laws, and programs. By doing this, the individual states can develop an understanding of how to best serve the needs of their populations. The people living in these states can have some type of treatment that was unthinkable twenty-one years ago.

While this list is remarkable, it also points out some current problems. It is important for each state to determine its own fate regarding medical cannabis, but basic rights of every citizen need to be secured. It is the role of the federal government to protect those rights. Many are still in jail and prison for personal use of cannabis. Every state that has medical cannabis laws on the books or pending has made its own determination about illnesses covered, allowable substances and embodiments, amounts allowed for personal possession, home cultivation, dispensary operation, and caregivers' rights to help the seriously ill patient. Unfortunately, this has led to widely variable laws and rights that leave people at risk even if they are following the law. It also forces people to lose significant treatment for themselves and their family members if they move from one state to another with different laws. The problem is that misconceptions remain about this treatment being all about CBD and THC, and that is just not the case. This is an ancient treatment we are just getting a better understanding of now. It has already proven itself to be safe, not just because there are minimal CB-1 receptors in life-support areas of the brain (brainstem), but because this plant is highly compatible with the endocannabinoid system found in every animal on the planet. This compatibility means that cannabis does not suppress the endocannabinoid system, enhancing it only enough to exert its effects, but not enough to cause problems throughout the body. Instead, it enhances the way the promiscuous endocannabinoid system works on itself and at least seven other major systems in the body to restore and maintain balance.

Limiting medical cannabis use to a predetermined CBD-to-THC ratio or specific legislated diseases limits the effectiveness of this treatment by restricting TCP and by limiting physicians from exploring where they feel this treatment might work. Some states have left a clause in the law that the treating physician can determine what should be treated, but most are much more restrictive. There is no medicine available that a physician is restricted from trying for a reason other than its intended use. Certainly, insurance companies often refuse to cover these uses, but the physician has the option to try things with patients. This is a good idea, because there are many cases of many illnesses that do not respond to anything standard, for which physicians need to provide other options. Use of medical cannabis delivers a whole new set of options, with its broad list of medically valuable cannabinoids. It also creates a genuine partnership between informed physicians and their patients to make choices, and turns over more control of care to the patient.

The other problematic restriction is with possession amounts. While the obvious attempt here is to limit the amount that people have in their possession to prevent a revitalization of the black market, this reasoning fails in the face of recommendations for the use of capsules with raw and heated plants, concentrated oil and flowers for vaporization, use of oral concentrates or smoked cannabis, hashish, or other concentrates. This variety of treatment and ability of people to make their own edible capsules, providing more controlled measurements and strain specificity, is an emerging treatment strategy, as delineated in this book. Specific restrictions of phytocannabinoids and of possession limits below several ounces greatly limit creative solutions to stubborn health problems. It also restricts treatment in some states for conditions that respond to variable and broad TCPs.

In addition to the above, the variability of this treatment in different states is as if a pharmaceutical had different limits and different routes of administration available in different states, and did not operate at all in others. The illness a person has in California is the same if the person vacations in Idaho. Yet that person cannot legally pursue that treatment in a different locale then where the treatment was established. This makes no sense for real medical care.

Medical cannabis treatment is mired in the image of it just being about THC or CBD, when it is really about THC, CBD, THCA, CBDA, THCV, CBC, CBN, CBG, CBDV, and another 102 cannabinoids, whose properties are still being figured out. It is also about the synergy between these substances based on their shifting ratios of one to the other. THC has excellent medical value. When this is removed from the list of treatment options, treatment success is likely to be more limited. The strategy to increase the TCP to achieve the best and longest-lasting outcome is thus eviscerated.

The result is that when people experience success or failure under these limited circumstances, it doesn't really mean anything about either. It just means that the scope of the treatment could not be entirely explored because the options are too limited.

This isn't even a matter of just controlling THC use. This type of policy eliminates other approaches, like THCA use through ingesting the raw plant or even an appropriate level of THCV. Complicating the problem further is that all these products can transform into one another long after they are harvested, they are refined, and their TCP is measured. Since these changes occur routinely, what is tested rarely turns out to be accurate in the long run. The ratios of cannabinoids and their absolute values constantly change. It is likely that this variation is one of the real advantages of this treatment, as explained earlier. Restricting any of it because of misconceived beliefs about the nature of the treatment is short-sighted. Since medical conditions are the same from state to state, this restrictive approach flies in the face of equal treatment for all, but that is still far better than no treatment for anyone.

In states with less restrictive laws for medical cannabis, chaos has not reigned. In California, the treatment is more extensively used than anywhere else in the country, with estimated users numbering more than 1,000,000 people. Despite this, California has seen no big increase in marijuana-related crime or deterioration of the social fabric. It's still a nice place to live. In my practice, because I have full access to this treatment, I have been able to use it on some of the worst persistent pain problems with outstanding success in reducing pain, improving function, and reducing pharmaceuticals. If I was limited to a CBD-only law, even one that allowed for the treatment of pain as most CBD-specific laws do not, success would be more muted.

Another problem with federal law is that different laws affect different aspects of how this treatment is allowed to grow and flourish or atrophy and whither. Banking and securities laws prevent the business aspects of medical cannabis from developing. It is against the law for banks to allow cannabis businesses to have bank accounts or invest in stocks, and other securities. Travel within the United States is highly restricted. There is no law against businesses firing those to be found with THC or other cannabinoids in urine or blood tests. The federal Centers for Disease Control (CDC) recommends in its Opioid Guidelines that testing for THC be removed from urine screens as a reason to eliminate opioid treatment to those who have this in their urine samples. However, this practice and its consequences continue.

It seems that one of the largest problems is the continued misunderstanding of this treatment, rooted in the lack of scientific exploration and information dissemination to the medical profession. Most physicians believe that medical cannabis treatment consists of smoking a joint and getting high. They do not have even a modest exposure to the endocannabinoid system and its far-reaching effects on maintaining balance and fighting chronic disease. This will certainly become part of the teaching in medical curricula, but it remains tainted by the misconception that the most common treatment is just about being stoned. In fact, it is about how to do this without getting stoned, if those effects are undesirable. Another issue is that physicians often certify, but do not treat the patient with medical cannabis. Physicians prescribe medications with standard doses and stable shelf lives. Treating with medical cannabis is different, because the substance changes constantly over time.

Unfortunately, patients also often think that the treatment is a failure if they are not feeling high. One of the main purposes of writing this book is to dispel this misinformation, and to look at this treatment as an evolving way to improve clinical outcomes by restoring balance in the body. It is also incredibly effective at altering the neuroplastic problems the brain develops secondary to the constant input of chronic illness. Medical cannabis can restore many of these neuroplastic changes back to normal. To be clear, this is not mere symptom management or suppression. This is actually disease resolution and restoration of normal function. While medical cannabis cannot heal all injured or damaged tissue, it can significantly improve the consequences caused by pervasive, negative neuroplastic change, by creating positive neuroplastic change, the goal of all effective treatment for chronic illnesses.

Understanding the versatility of this treatment is important for people in positions to determine public policy. While voters can approve or disapprove medical cannabis laws, state legislators determine how these laws will be structured. This has a huge influence on effectiveness of any treatment. Often legislators are poorly informed about the scope of this treatment option, and believe there is efficacy for medical cannabis treatment for specific conditions. This is not determined. It cannot be determined until physicians are free to prescribe specific strains and embodiments of the plant to take advantage of the various TCPs, routes of administration, absorption rates, and elimination dynamics, in order to make thoughtful recommendations. Training of physicians is important, but no more so than thoughtful input to state legislators about the treatment itself. Additionally, the public should be informed about the potential effects, that this treatment is not just about getting high, and that it can in fact be conducted quite well without getting high at all. Any treatment that works around the clock should not alter consciousness, if it is to be a viable option. Even if a person enjoys the feeling of being high, treatment with medical cannabis cannot be effective if that person has to be stoned on a constant basis.

In summary, state laws are variable and serve to provide access to treatment with medical cannabis in substantially different ways. Some of the problem is that no overarching federal law, other than complete illegality of cannabis or any phytocannabinoid exists. This law is in conflict with those developed by states. The current "don't ask don't tell" agreements do nothing significant to rectify this issue and will have to be resolved in the future. While states with medical cannabis laws do provide access, they do not provide for continuity of care from one part of the country to another. This is not a way to allow for a person receiving successful treatment in Colorado to move or vacation in any other state and continue this treatment for their serious medical condition. There is no medical treatment in traditional medicine that has these types of restrictions. The first hurdle to overcome is that of the misunderstanding that this treatment is about smoking a joint and getting high. This misconception is held by legislators, physicians and the public. Second, the idea of restricting physician recommendations to specific conditions that vary from state to state, is nonsense and flies in the face of the basic principles of medical care of providing accessible, coordinated and quality health care to all people. Third, legislators in states need to have access to more rational education about this substance and its potential medical utility. This information needs to be extended to the public at large, in order to dispel the myths that surround medical cannabis treatment and to remove the stigma of users of this care being "stoners." Finally, and perhaps of greatest importance, is for the development of deeper understanding and training for physicians and medical students about the workings of the endocannabinoid system and effective treatment with medical cannabis.

Chapter 8

Grow Your Own Medicine

THIS CHAPTER TITLE SHOULD NOT be taken literally. While there are ideas about growing cannabis, this section also will look at how to transform that cannabis into tinctures, capsules, food additives, and topicals. It will also explore cooperative growing and recommend a few ideas for the user of medical cannabis to establish a dedicated grower. This chapter will also discuss the advantages of indoor and outdoor growing. However, it is not meant as directions for growing; rather, it is a general description about growing for individual patients seeking to decrease the expense of this treatment, and to grow and process the precise strains and phytocannabinoid profiles they seek. There are books and websites written and available on the details of this, and I will not go into the specifics of how cannabis is grown. One of the hidden aspects of medical cannabis treatment is that it is enjoyable, not only because of pleasant psychotropic effects from THC, but also in the act of working out the details of individual treatment plans and seeing them come to fruition over time. Nowhere is this more apparent than in growing and transforming the plant into various treatment modalities.

Growing cannabis is steeped in traditions developed over time. Everyone who grows this plant has their own special touch they bring to the process. Some of these are common and time-honored, but may not be necessary. They do, however, establish a ritual rhythm to growing these plants, and a new grower should explore as many of these growing techniques as feasible, to become more comfortable with the process and develop one's own pattern, rhythms, and rituals. Everyone who grows has strongly held beliefs about what is best. Many work as well as each other, and finding one's own comfort zone will probably yield the best results. Be open to tips from others who are more experienced, and experiment as you go on by keeping good written records of each grow.

Cannabis is not a weed, even though "weed" is a slang term used to describe it. It is, however, a hardy plant, with beautiful flower structures and a clear vegetative and flowering stage of growth. Plants can be grown from seeds, but these are hard to find, expensive, and uncertain. Once procured, they can be planted in a flower pot, outdoors in soil in the spring, and will vegetate during the summer, finally flowering in the fall. Many strains grow quite tall in this environment. Given its distinctive leaves, this can make cannabis highly conspicuous. Even in legal states, this to be avoided in favor of more discreet, secure approaches. One such approach is to grow indoors, but this is more complicated than growing house plants or growing cannabis outdoors.

EQUIPMENT

Generally, it takes special equipment to achieve a harvest of flowering plants with an indoor grow. This can be quite expensive or, with a more DIY spirit, rather inexpensive. The most important factor for growing good cannabis is light, and the type and timing of light used is a critical factor determining success or failure. The total amount of light determines when cannabis flowers. One of the advantages of growing it indoors is that with the right equipment, the grower can control this variable. The result is faster flowering and often more perfect-looking flowers than can be grown outdoors. That is not to say that the quality of outdoor grown plants is not as good or better than indoors, but cosmetics probably favor skilled indoor-grown plants. Light types vary, with standard lighting tending to be fluorescent, metal halide (MH), high-pressure sodium (HPS), and light emitting diode (LED). High-output fluorescent lights put out more light than normal fluorescent lights, and different color spectra can be substituted for vegetative and flowering stages. Fluorescents run much cooler than the MH or HPS lights, and tend to need less elaborate cooling ducts and exhaust fans, depending on the indoor garden type. MH and HPS are good options, but their heat output and electricity use are much higher than other lights'. Heat output is important because plants have ideal heat ranges for their growth, and too much heat will cause problems and lower yields. These lights can be used in different stages of growing the plant. LEDs are the most expensive lighting option in initial cost, but tend to run the coolest and use the least electricity. They too require less extensive cooling ducts and exhaust fans.

GROWING CANNABIS

Cannabis is a dioecious plant, meaning that it has male and female forms. It is the female form that has the most abundant cannabinoids, and keeping the male and female segregated during flowering prevents pollination and seed formation. This stimulates the cannabinoids to concentrate in the flowers and leaves of the female plant, evidenced by glandular structures called trichomes forming on the flowers and leaves. The greatest concentration of trichomes is on the stamens in the flowers of the female plant.

Cannabis goes through stages of growth like most flowering or fruiting plants. There is a germinating stage, a vegetative stage, and a flowering stage. Cannabis can also be grown from clones of plants, leading to a greater (but not guaranteed) consistency of phytocannabinoid components. Fifty to a hundred generations can be cloned until a fresh plant grown from seed is necessary to use. The seedling takes about seven to ten days to germinate, and this is determined by the formation of roots. Clones can be in light 18 to 24 hours. Once this happens, the plants can be transplanted into another small pot to let them make a transition to vegetation.

This first transitional phase requires 18 to 24 hours of light, which is extended from the transitional phase to vegetative phase. This takes another week or two, and can be extended if necessary. Clones can be kept in a state of suspended animation if placed in a gallon plastic bag, in their small pot or net cup, with a small amount of 1/4 strength growth type of nutrients and sealed. They will survive without any significant growth for several months in this condition. Once you are ready, the plant can be transplanted to a larger pot (soil) or net cup (hydroponics). Then, allow this to vegetate with proper nutrients, anywhere from three to four weeks to two months. If growing indoors, the time is shorter; outdoors it is longer. In indoor grows, when vegetating plants are healthy and strong, and have grown to about 1/3 the distance to the top of the grow space, they can be switched to flowering by changing the nutrients and lighting. Nutrients are switched to blooming flowers, but vegetative growth continues, with the plant attaining two or three times the size it was when flowering begins. Pre-packaged nutrients for the various stages of plant growth are freely available at nursery and hydroponic stores. In the flowering stage, lights are now changed to 12 hours on and 12 hours off. Indoor grown plants take a few weeks to go through a transition and begin to flower. These will continue to do so, and as long as not pollinated by a male plant, the plants will develop glands called trichomes on the flowers. This is where the highest concentration of the phytocannabinoids will develop. As the trichomes mature they will also develop on leaves in close proximity to the flowers. When these flowers reach full maturity, it will be time to harvest the plants and dry and cure them. Finally, the flowers are trimmed and the buds are cured. Leaves can be saved and used fresh in food or dried and used like the flowers. While they won't have the potency of the flowers, they will have their own phytocannabinoid profile, and can add to the TCP and the variability of treatment, which is the goal of the advanced medical cannabis therapy.

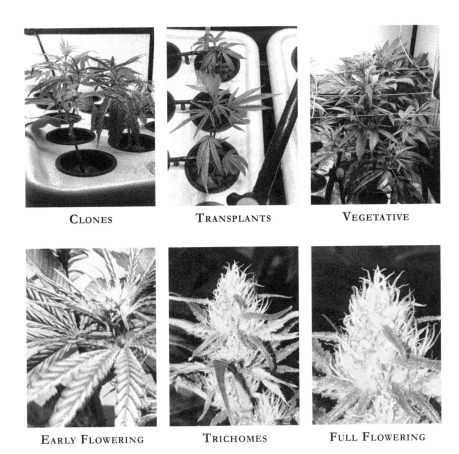

CLONES   TRANSPLANTS   VEGETATIVE

EARLY FLOWERING   TRICHOMES   FULL FLOWERING

Outdoor growing is quite different, because once plants are vegetating, they depend on the length of the day for their transition from vegetation to flowering. They generally take longer then indoor-grown plants, but also tend to grow much larger. They are more susceptible to degradation through various large and microscopic creatures, but tend to be quite hardy with proper tending. They will also give larger yields of higher phytocannabinoid concentrations than indoor grown plants, although indoor growing is usually close in concentration of cannabinoids to outdoor growing. The risk of stray pollination is low, as long as male plants are removed when they first flower and the plants are not growing in an area with a high density of outdoor cannabis gardens. Male plants are easily identified from female plants when flowering begins, and there are several weeks of flowering of these plants before they produce pollen. Bees and birds do not spread the male pollen, although wind does so. Good management of indoor grows can control all variables, including light, air circulation, nutrients, soil, and hydroponics. That does not mean that success is guaranteed, as practice tends to improve technique and grow quality and quantity. Soil is generally easier to grow in than hydroponics, but hydroponic growing is very efficient and can be dialed into the exact desired nutrients, pH and parts per million (PPM) required for best results. Humidity and temperature can be controlled. Carbon dioxide can be infused into the growth area during light times, if desired, but exhaust fans need to be shut off during these infusions. Outdoor growing depends on Mother Nature and the specifics of climate in the grow region. This leaves a lot more to chance, but results can be spectacular and surprisingly consistent. Usually, outdoor grows are much friendlier to the environment, leaving a smaller carbon footprint, than comparable indoor grows.

This varies based on how high-tech the growing space is and how much electricity it uses. It also depends on the skill and experience of the grower

PRUNING

Pruning the plant is also helpful. The idea is to prune the leaves that are blocked from the light, to decrease the energy being devoted to the substructure of the plant. Here the goal is to open up space and to have enough light shine through that the whole plant is exposed to it. As the canopy thickens and covers lower branches, an alternative to pruning is bending and tying down the upper crown of the plant to expose more of the flowers to the light. This also helps the plant continue to grow in indoor space that it is outgrowing. Some people top off the flowers in the canopy to get a larger yield, because two flowers will replace the one that is topped off. Some even recommend leaving a small nub of the flower in place for even better yield. Lollipopping the plant takes the lower branches and prunes away the side leaves supporting the growth nodes that will become or are already early flowers. This results in the flowering part of the plant growing up from the lower part of it into the canopy for best light and higher yield.

Good books on the subject are everywhere. Two excellent ones are *Marijuana Horticulture: The Indoor/Outdoor Medical Grower's Bible* by Jorge Cervantes and *Marijuana Grower's Handbook* by Ed Rosenthal. These are both quite comprehensive and very helpful grower's guides. More general books on gardening and hydroponics are also good resources.

Furthermore, the internet is a source of written and video information that can be useful in growing cannabis. An excellent web resource is growweedeasy.com. This website is especially helpful to correct growing mistakes or to prepare for the next stage of your own growing experience. Be aware that everyone who grows cannabis has their own ideas about what is correct or even essential. These are pretty hardy and forgiving plants, and with a modicum of care, they will grow rather robustly. Critical errors in growing tend to occur a lot more frequently when obsessing over proper growth technique. It is important to take the time and be open to some failures or shortfalls, so that these can be corrected. Even indoor grows can become infested with spider mites and mold, so having good written references can be invaluable in both detecting and dealing with problems in all stages of the grow.

HARVEST

Once the plant flowers, the question is when to harvest. Some recommendations are to harvest the indoor strain female plants one to three weeks after bud formation slows. Others are to look at the trichomes on the flowers with a handheld magnifying device. These resin glands change from clear to milky to amber. A week prior to harvesting the both indoor and outdoor grown plants should be flushed with a nutrient solution designed to provide the plants with nutrition, but to clean it out of fertilizer, so that taste is improved. There is no danger that this presents to consumption if this step is skipped, but the experience of smoking or vaporizing will be smoother if the plants are flushed prior to harvest.

Cervantes recommends harvesting *Cannabis sativa* varieties when resin glands are mostly clear and a few are milky white. Harvesting *Cannabis indica* varieties are best when the resin glands turn amber.[133] Others feel that both should not be harvested until at least 50% of the trichomes are milky and some amber trichomes are showing up. The biggest mistake is of harvesting too early. The plants are harvested by cutting the stem at the soil or hydroponic net cup line, and then hanging them in a dark place to dry them. The large leaves are best trimmed before drying the plant, because they are more difficult to remove when dry. It is completely unnecessary to hang the plants upside down, although this may be a convenient way to dry them. The resin of the plants will not flow to the flowers

---

133   Cervantes J, *Marijuana Horticulture: The Indoor/Outdoor Medical Growers Bible* (Vancouver, B.C., Van Patten Publishing, 2006): 79–84.

if one does this. Once a plant is harvested, it will no longer produce any more phytocannabinoids, but will continue to change the ratios of these until the last fragment of it is consumed. They should be trimmed at the stem to prevent mold, while the plants are drying. There are other drying devices on the market. The idea is to dry the flowers and leaves evenly. Once dried, plants can be hand-trimmed. There are also electric trimmers and trimming machines, but these are best saved for people growing larger crops. Saving the trim is a good idea, as it will have a different phytocannabinoid profile than the flowers, and can be used in making capsules, tinctures, and hashish.

DRYING AND CURING

Once the plant is dried (usually a week at 60–70° Fahrenheit (15–21° Celsius) and 40–60% humidity, it needs to be trimmed, then cured. Trimming is best done over a trimming station with a screen over the upper part to catch the falling resin in the lower half. There are numerous commercial products on the market.

Trimming is done with scissors. This is time-consuming and considered unpleasant by growers, but essential to selling clean cannabis flowers. For home growers, the process is a lot more pleasant, because they are not trimming pounds of buds, usually. As with everything else in growing this plant, there are numerous opinions about the correct way to cure the plant. A simple way is to put the dried plant in a turkey or goose bag and throw in a torn-up tortilla with it to absorb and contribute moisture. A time-honored approach is to put it in a cool dark area in mason jars, opening to the air once or twice daily for a few weeks. Some people cure the plant for months, but this is probably overkill. For plants high in CBD, traditional methods are followed for curing.

TINCTURES

Although the cured plant can be smoked or vaporized, it can easily be made into either alcohol or oil-based tinctures, as well. The advantage of tinctures is that they are swallowed, allowing them a longer period of activity in the bloodstream and in bodily tissues than smoked or vaporized material. Another great advantage is that they can be slowly raised and lowered, drop by drop. This makes for a safe way to determine what is tolerable, while exploring effectiveness.

Oil-based tinctures are usually made with olive oil, but can be made with other oils, such as coconut oil or sesame seed oil. The traditional way of making tinctures is to decarboxylate the plant by heating it in an oven at 250 to 300 degrees for an hour, then crumbling in by hand into olive oil. One ounce of cannabis for 8 fluid ounces of olive oil is the general proportion. When the plant is decarboxylated the acid forms of phytocannabinoids are transformed into the non-acid forms. This activates THCA to THC and CBDA to CBD. The olive oil/cannabis mixture is heated then for 4 hours on a low setting in a slow cooker. It is cooled for another hour, then filtered through a cheesecloth followed by a second filtering with a coffee filter. Plant matter is separated. Some wrap the cheesecloth into a poultice to be used over aching areas on the body. This can be frozen to cool the skin while body temperature warms and releases the cannabinoids. Others just throw it out. Alcohol-based tincture requires a high-proof alcohol, such as 151 proof rum or 190 proof Everclear. 151 proof Everclear is also useful and in a pinch Vodka can be a useful tincture vehicle. The plants are decarboxylated, as above, and then one hand-ground ounce is put in 32 fluid ounces of the alcohol and shaken up. It is stored in a cool dark place such as the freezer. The alcohol mixture is shaken every day for a month to two months, and the tincture is refined similarly to the olive oil-based product: through cheesecloth first, then a coffee filter.

Another technique is to use a device designed to make tinctures, such as the Magical Butter. This resembles an electric coffee pot, but has a macerating blade inside that turns on and off during the 4-8-hour heating cycle to grind up the pre-heated plant matter. This allows for extraction of the phytocannabinoids from the plant, which dissolve into the alcohol. This does not require one to two months of shaking up the mixture and allows for immediate consumption when done. The Magical Butter also can be used to make tincture in oil and to make cooking butter or oil.

Once the cannabis is made into an alcohol-based tincture, it can be ingested or it can be altered by letting the alcohol evaporate and allowing the tincture to dry on the bottom and side of a heat-resistant glass container. One teaspoon of olive oil can be added, and the bottom and side residue can be stirred into it, creating a concentrate cannabis oil. This is a far safer way of doing this than using solvents other than alcohol. Evaporation is also a much safer way to make concentrate than by using an open flame or even electrical heating.

EAT IT RAW

Juicing the plant is also an option, but requires fresh plant, and a great deal of it. A compromise is to save the pruned leaves and freshly harvested leaves in a plastic bag in the refrigerator, using them raw in smoothies. This allows use of the raw plant, and incorporates the acid forms of phytocannabinoids into the diet. The result is a broader TCP.

MAKING TOPICALS

Cannabis tincture can be added to various lotions or can be the active ingredient in body creams or body butters. This is another way of using higher-THC forms of the plant, without psychotropic effects. This can also combine various ratios of tinctures made from high-CBD and high-THC plants, as well as specialized cannabinoid tinctures high in THCA or THCV or THCVA. These lotions can have a profound effect on local pain.

Making Capsules

Making capsules requires a grinder and the other material. That grinder could be a hand-held shredder, but an inexpensive dedicated electric coffee grinder is better and will grind cannabis more finely. It can also grind other substances, such as raw cacao nibs, turmeric, or cayenne. Combining all ingredients in the coffee grinder makes for the best blending process, as well. For combined components, the following are reasonable techniques.

Table 17: Customized Advanced Medical Cannabis Treatment

Capsule Blend	Technique
Cannabis + Raw Cacao **Cannabis + Tumeric** **Cannabis + Cayenne**	1. Grind cannabis in the coffee grinder raw high THC and/or after pre-heated in oven for one hour at 300 degrees >20:1 CBD:THC 2. Grind raw cacao nibs in coffee grinder. Add t tsp tumeric or 1/4 tsp cayenne 3. Measure equal amounts of both for a 50/50 mix or more or less depending on individual dosing desire 4. Put both amounts of plant and cacao back into grinder and grind together 5. Stuff into "00" sized capsules

Capsule Blend	Technique
Cannabis + Raw cacao + Tumeric + Cayanne	1. Grind cannabis in the coffee grinder raw high THC and/or after pre-heated in oven for one hour at 300 degrees >20:1 CBD:THC 2. Grind raw cacao nibs in coffee grinder 3. Add 1/4 tsp of Cayenne and 1 tsp of Tumeric to cacao nibs and grind 4. Measure equal amounts of both for a 50/50 mix or more or less depending on individual dosing desire 5. Put both amounts of plant and cacao, cayenne, Tumeric blend back into grinder and grind together 6. Stuff into "00" sized capsules
Cannabis + GABA	1. Grind cannabis in the coffee grinder raw high THC and/or after pre-heated in oven for one hour at 300 degrees >20:1 CBD:THC 2. Measure out cannabis and add equal amounts of GABA for a 50/50 mix or more or less depending on individual dosing desire 3. Grind together briefly 4. Stuff into "00" sized capsules

Capsules can be made with cooked or raw plant, and each presents its own advantages. The raw plant is not as likely to cause a psychoactive response, so using it this way is one of the ways to use medical cannabis with far less risk of having these effects. The broadest phytocannabinoid profile is accomplished by combining raw and cooked plants. It is best to make these into separate capsules that can be stored in labeled bottles so that they can be taken at appropriate time with predictable effects. As always, these should be tested when there is plenty of free time for the effects to wear off, before assuming that they will not cause psychotropic effects. Capsules can be made for each strain or several strains can be combined, further customizing and sculpting the treatment.

TESTING

Testing is also highly recommended, but it can be costly, so this is certainly optional. Finding a local lab that can test what you grow will let you know aspects of the TCP, but it will not cover all cannabinoids, and what it does cover will shift over time. Still it will give you a good idea of where you are starting, and the changes are not necessarily going to be dramatic, although effects over time may change. Some labs will give the phytocannabinoid profile of all of the medicinal cannabinoids, but at the least should give CBDA, CBD, THCA and THC levels.

STORAGE

Storing the cannabis in a humidity-controlled environment can be very helpful. As stated in the Paraphernalia Chapter of this book, Boveda makes packets that are designed to keep cannabis stable and fresh at 62% humidity. This can be most easily accomplished by throwing the appropriate sized Boveda packet into a mason jar with the stored plant or in another product called the C-Vault. The C-Vault comes in various sizes, and has a built-in storage area for the Boveda packet in its lid. A humidor is another option, but specialized cannabis humidors are a first choice. They do not use the traditional Spanish cedar found in cigar humidors, instead using neutral-smelling wood, such as mahogany. This is covered more extensively in the Paraphernalia chapter.

Cooperative or Dedicated Growing

In states that allow cooperative or dedicated growers, people may find them an easy, far less expensive way to secure their particular strains, than purchasing from a dispensary. Commercial growers will grow what brings in the most money. Rarely, some will seek to grow plants with specific medical traits. This will certainly occur more frequently in the future, but the problem will remain that supply will always seek to match demand, and the demand for recreational cannabis will always outstrip the demand for medical cannabis. The problem of supply of specific strains can be achieved by cooperative and designated growing. A cooperative group can select a grower to grow specific plants to meet medical needs. These plants could include high-CBD and low-THC, even ratios of CBD and THC, high-THC and low-CBD, specific strains to combine effects, or specialized plants high in THCV and CBG. This type of cooperative agreement could allow the consumer to dedicate and purchase a whole plant to be grown by an experienced grower. The grower would receive payment for several plants, determining with the co-op members which strains they wish to have grown. Cost would be based on whole plants, not finished and trimmed buds. The co-op members would perform the task of determining which members would receive specific plants. Any embodiments would be made by the co-op members solely for their own use. In this way, the risk and cost are spread out, the grower receives a fair price, and the consumer can get a palette of plants that can cover their health needs in a planned manner. The other obvious advantages are that an experienced grower can deliver very high-quality plants to the co-op, and guarantee they are organic and pesticide-free.

To grow one's own medicine is a deeply satisfying experience. When this saves money and lets the user make their own embodiments, it just gets better. Medical cannabis is a treatment that, by law, is not supported by any health insurance. This means it is an expense above and beyond traditional medical care. Because medical cannabis is not a replacement for traditional medical care, its added cost is not insignificant. Perhaps this is the reason that in states where medical cannabis is legal, use of pharmaceuticals that can be substituted with medical cannabis decreased by 25%. Certainly, compared to the cost of pharmaceuticals, medical cannabis is a bargain, but insurance pays a substantial amount of their cost in most situations. The best way to offset that extra expense is for patients to grow their own cannabis in the states where this is legal.

Beyond the issues of cost, there is the issue of strain availability. Growing the specific strains needed are the best way to guarantee supplies. For those who live in states that allow for cooperative and/or designated growing, these avenues can be economical and species-specific. Once the plant is growing, there are many resources available to help it grow, and those who grow their own cannabis report it is a genuinely satisfying experience. Some feel it is a spiritual activity, far more meaningful than growing other plants. Others describe the pleasure of treating their conditions with something that they have brought forth from the earth. Regardless, the opportunity to participate in one's own care in selecting, growing, refining, experimenting, and planning is rare in today's medical culture of short visits, physician-directed care, and patient passivity. While growing the plant takes patience and energy, the rewards are far greater than consuming what is grown.

In summary, growing specific plants either indoors or outdoors can be a means of having a less expensive supply of specific strains that can lead to a selected TCP tailored to the individual patient's needs. This not only allows for a decrease in cost of this treatment, but involves the patient in an active means of controlling their own medical conditions, while enjoying the experience of growing and preparing their treatment. This is only available to patients in states that allow growing for personal use. If growing areas are not available or if use of more experienced cultivators is desirable, designated growers can grow plants for individuals and co-ops, again if state law allows. It is always important to make sure of the local legality of this activity.

Epilogue

SINCE I STARTED WRITING THIS book, much has changed in the world. Regardless of these changes, in the United States and more and more of the world, the medicinal value of medical cannabis is an established fact of life. Millions of people use this for treatment, and they are not walking around stoned, nor are they going to walk away from treatment with medical cannabis. These are responsible people seeking to play a meaningful role in managing their own health issues. This movement started with the people who believed it was helpful from personal experience and that of family members, and it grew dramatically popular over the last two decades, to the point that forty-four states and the District of Columbia have legalized the use of cannabis in some form for some conditions.

Physicians, charged with certifying patients for this treatment, have largely stayed on the sidelines, citing the need for more evidence before they could endorse it. They are one of the main reasons I have written this book. One of the major issues for physicians to understand is that this is a relatively safe treatment with no lethal dose. It is also one that is very different than usual medical care, in that it requires a great deal of patient experimentation, and would benefit tremendously from physicians helping guide patients, rather than directing them. Furthermore, this treatment is steeped in excellent science, published in the best peer-reviewed journals in the world. There is no lack of scientific or pharmacological evidence of the efficacy of cannabis and the phytocannabinoids. There are small randomized, double-blind, placebo-controlled trials (RCTs), but none of these can or will ever be able to determine if medical cannabis is an effective treatment for any condition. That is like looking for an RCT to prove that pills work for inflammation. Some do, some don't and some make inflammation worse. The same is likely to be true for medical cannabis, which is a different treatment with different strains, embodiments, and routes of administration. What stimulates appetite (THC) is not helpful for someone with a gastric bypass or sleeve type of weight loss surgery, but it can be quite effective for chemotherapy-induced or cancer-induced wasting problems. CBD, which promotes weight loss, would need to be balanced with some THC to offset its weight-losing qualities.

A better way to look at this treatment, scientifically, involves the collection of big data and of individual practice data. Currently, we are building an application to collect these data and to make them available to physicians, on both the larger scale of all patients participating in the data-collection aspect of our app and the smaller scale of patients participating in physicians' own individual practices. Another important concept is that the synergistic effects of the various phytocannabinoids adding up to much more than the sum of the parts. Even when several phytocannabinoids result in the same effect (anti-inflammatory, analgesic, anti-tumor), they all achieve this by working on different aspects of endocannabinoid and several other systems in the body. Furthermore, the endocannabinoid system and the phytocannabinoid system should be seen not as blockers or enhancers, but as modulators of many basic somatic systems that together work to restore balance and normal function. As such, they may take some time to work, but when they do, both systems can help restore normal health, function, and wellbeing. A good example is weight loss using high-CBD cannabis. This may take three to six months to show an effect, but once it happens, not only is white fat turned into brown fat, but there is a slowly developing positive effect on hypothalamic satiety centers. Weight loss occurs because of the former, but satiation occurs much earlier in a meal, as well. This results in nearly effortless loss of weight for many, with the pounds just pouring off, then stabilizing. There is currently no known pharmacologic or non-pharmacologic weight loss treatment that does anything like this.

The best place for physicians to start with medical cannabis treatment is to gain an understanding of the endocannabinoid system. The chapter on endocannabinoids in this book is designed as a way to gain a quick but deep understanding of this system. It is well documented, but one should remember that as of this writing, a PubMed search of *endocannabinoid* finds 8,835 peer-reviewed articles. By the time this book is published it will likely top 9,000 scientific articles on the endocannabinoid system. Additionally, there are currently 5,071 PubMed articles on medical cannabis. The vast majority of these combined 13,000 scientific articles on these two topics have been published in the last decade. Needless to say, independent research of this cornucopia of medical literature can be quite rewarding. It is highly recommended that physicians become more knowledgeable and therefore more helpful to their patients, about this type of treatment. Even if a physician never intends to use medical cannabis with their patients, understanding the workings of the endocannabinoid system unlocks the mysteries of wellness and health, due to its central roles in determining pleasure in the hedonic centers of the brain and its ability to nudge the body's multiple systems back toward normal by modulating multiple systems in the body.

This is why treatment with phytocannabinoids is skewed toward a positive result. Unlike pharmaceuticals, plant-based cannabinoids enhance and restore the system they work on, rather than suppressing and replacing it. Additionally, through 5,000 years of epigenetic experience, not only have humans altered the plant's genome, but the plant has altered ours. Even if a person has never tried marijuana, it is a substance that has changed their genome.

Perhaps the largest issue of all with medical cannabis for physician-guided treatment is its ability to decrease or replace medications, including opioids, to treat pain. This is about far more than just replacing opioids. Cannabis changes the synergies of the endocannabinoid system, the vanilloid system, the PPARγ system, the catecholamine system, the endorphin system, the GABA/glutamate system, the hypothalamic-pituitary-adrenal axis, and the immune system. No matter what other science is illuminated about the phytocannabinoids, this astounding fact is completely unique to the endocannabinoid and phytocannabinoid system, making it imperative to study these effects. Clearly, it is this balancing issue that makes it so effective in optimizing and even stopping pharmaceuticals, restoring many of them to temporary stopgap treatments that work better than as long-term treatments. It is the restoration of normal homeostasis, the body's system of checks and balances, that makes this both an extremely attractive potential treatment and an effective way to curtail pharmaceuticals that cannot restore normality because of their tendency to suppress and replace the systems they work on. While patients will not necessarily be able to replace all their pharmaceuticals, this treatment could help reduce these to the lowest useful dose. This has certainly been the experience of my practice. To reduce other medications safely, the guidance of one's physician is essential. This guidance will be largely absent, however, unless the treating physician is knowledgeable about medical cannabis as a treatment option. In my practice, as relayed to me by my patients, I have heard some of the smartest physicians I know deny recommendations of this treatment with the most ignorant of ideas, steeped in superstition, hearsay, and personal bias, not science. It would be far better for a physician to profess an ignorance about the subject than to fall back on the safety net of "a lack of evidence," which is false at its core.

Then there is the issue of legality. Physicians who participate in this care, by certifying and advising their patients are currently protected by an act of Congress that makes state medical cannabis laws primary and federal laws secondary in states that have legalized medical cannabis as a treatment option. This was affirmed again in the 2017 congressional budget agreement, which makes it clear that the Justice Department is to allow states to determine their own cannabis laws, including recreational laws. Again, this passed with bipartisan support. It is abundantly clear that one of the only issues that appears to unify liberals and conservatives is the appropriate availability of medical cannabis for treatment. Physicians who participate in this treatment and follow state laws are protected. It would behoove participating physicians to review state law and state medical board interpretation of these laws. Physicians are not being prosecuted for recommending medical cannabis to their patients, as long as they follow their state laws.

Finally, a situation that must cease is the elimination of other treatment for those using medical cannabis. This is a problem perpetuated by the myth that if a patient is taking medical cannabis, they should be prevented from taking any schedule 2 drugs. Again, it is critical for physicians to understand that the current law is clear: in states with medical cannabis laws, those laws take precedence over federal law. Pain practitioners often discharge patients who are found to have THC in their urine toxicology screen. There is no real scientific rationale for this. Even the CDC's very strict opioid prescribing guidelines advise physicians to remove THC from urine testing, and warns that if doctors discharge patients from treatment based on positive findings of THC in the urine, this could be construed as patient abandonment. Ultimately, physicians have complete control over this issue, but the ethical problems are clear. Eliminating patients from other care because they have THC in their urine should not be a blanket policy of a practice or individual practitioner, and needs to be evaluated on a case-by-case basis, as should any other type of medical treatment.

Patients must understand this treatment does not require a person to feel high to be effective. There cannot be a legitimate medical treatment that leaves the person using it impaired all the time. Medical cannabis is a treatment that can be used without ever feeling high, although this should not be a deal breaker. There is always a risk of the unintended effect of any treatment, and the cognitive altering and psychotropic effects of medical cannabis treatment are no exception. Having said this, careful planning and use of appropriate strains, embodiments, and routes of administration can account for effective, safe, and stable treatment, without fear of being altered in inappropriate situations. This calls for a fair amount of self-experimentation in relatively safe situations to determine what is altering and what is not.

Safety must be a first priority with medical cannabis treatment. This includes keeping cannabis and paraphernalia for its use in a secure environment if living with children or if they are visiting. For younger children, this is to prevent accidental ingestion; for adolescents, it is about securing it from illegal use and diversion. There is a movement among pharmacists and physicians to keep meds safe by keeping them in a secure and locked box to avoid these issues. This should also be applied to medical cannabis.

There is also the issue of driving under the influence. This is the same risk as with other potentially psychotropic medications. If a user is stopped and tested, it is the judgment call of the officer involved that determines a DUI arrest and filing of charges. In a treatment that occurs around the clock, there is no way of avoiding the risk of a bad call by the police, resulting in a socially stigmatizing, costly, and risky legal situation. On the other hand, using high-CBD, low-THC strains during the day and saving higher-THC strains after driving is done for the day is a wiser, safer way to use this treatment. The law on this subject will develop over the next several years, and, hopefully clear parameters will be established, but this will take some time.

It is also important to monitor other medications being used in the face of high-CBDA or CBD cannabis, which can alter the way other medications are accumulated or eliminated. If symptoms or side effects from these medications emerge, speaking to one's primary-care physician is essential to adjust treatment dosing with these medications. Usually, a simple adjustment will work. Most interactions are theoretical and unlikely to be clinically significant. On the other hand, everyone is different. That fact shows the importance of working in partnership with one's physician to manage this treatment. Physicians should determine if they are comfortable or not with making a recommendation for medical cannabis, but discomfort with the recommendation is not a reason to reject this treatment for their patient. As with any area of expertise that crosses the threshold of individual physician comfort, if the physician does not feel they can make a competent recommendation, a referral to someone who can evaluate the situation should be the course of action. If a physician tells a patient that this treatment is too risky because of there not being enough studies on this subject or enough clinical studies, you may politely ask for a consultation with a local physician who has experience with this treatment. Hopefully, this book will be of some benefit.

When physician and patient do collaborate, this treatment works best. Unlike traditional medical care, cannabis care should involve patient-based exploration of various strains, embodiments, and routes of administration. The patient should discuss with their treating physician the results of this self-experimentation, so that both patient and physician can learn together what works best for the patient. This also opens a forum for patient and physician to evaluate success and failure, side effects, drug interactions, and strategies for dealing with untoward psychotropic effects. Even if a physician has no training in treating with medical cannabis, their understanding of the patient's general health, and social issues is invaluable.

The best use of medical cannabis involves the mixing and matching of strains, embodiments, and routes of administration. There are infinite strains of cannabis available on the open market, but only one strain currently available from NIDA, the National Institute for Drug Abuse. This strain does not even begin to resemble the strains commonly available at dispensaries or grown by home growers. Among recreational users, the term *government-grade cannabis* is an ironic joke, indicating that the quality is low.

To NIDA's credit, it has put out a request for information (RFI) to the research community about strains, and embodiments regarding research experience. It has received and posted recommendations, which are not only reasonable but quite forward-thinking, at https://www.drugabuse.gov/drugs-abuse/marijuana/nidas-role-in-providing-marijuana- research/summary-request-information-rfi-regarding-varieties-marijuana-marijuana-products-research.

If NIDA does institute these recommendations, including growing and making available a wide variety of strains, potencies, biological extracts, and pure extracts, as well as evaluating drug interactions and disease specific effects, science should significantly benefit. One area that would be particularly useful is that of evaluating the efficacy of using marijuana to help people in pain get down and off opioids. This highlights the need to test multiple strains with different phytocannabinoid profiles, but testing must go beyond this, and include studying the effects of combining strains that are preheated and raw. NIDA's proposal also takes a look at different cannabis embodiments from oil-based tinctures to CO_2-extracted phytocannabinoid concentrates.

Until the research this policy promises to encourage is completed and analyzed, the current best practice is for the patient to mix and match various strains and to use several embodiments and routes of administration in the course of the day. These embodiments would include flowers, olive oil-based tinctures, alcohol-based tinctures, edibles, cannabis oil, hashish, preheated and unheated flowers ground and put into capsules, smoked, vaped, creams, and suppositories. The routes of administration would include swallowing, rubbing onto gums, inhalation, rectal, topical, intravaginal, and nasal. When looking at the infinite ways this type of treatment can be varied, it is easy to understand why declaring what form of medical cannabis can treat a specific medical condition is not accurate. While it may treat a specific condition in some people, it will not in others. Considering the variability, the real questions to be asked are about which strains, forms, and delivery methods have positive subjective and objective effects, and what happens when these approaches are combined and ultimately rotated? How do we deliver effective relief of symptoms and promotion of health and wellbeing, while minimizing side effects? When are psychotropic effects side effects, and when are they helpful or pleasurable? Since pleasurable experience is a driver of neuroplastic change, is this a way that cannabis evokes these changes? Can an individual match his or her own symptoms to several strains, embodiments, and routes of administration to take down symptoms and help restore health? It is in finding the answers to these questions that treatment with medical cannabis can be successful. There is little consistency in this treatment from person to person, which is what makes this treatment personalized to individual response.

Phytocannabinoid variability is based on the genetics of the plant, the environment it is planted in, the hours of sunlight the plant receives, the breeze that runs through a garden, and other factors. Just as each plant has its own scent, the phytocannabinoid profile of each plant is different from each other plant. Even if a cannabis plant is the same strain as the one next to it in the garden, it can have a significantly different phytocannabinoid profile. Using two different strains creates an even broader variability of phytocannabinoids. If these are grown indoors or outdoors or in two different parts of the same city the TCP will vary even more. The point is that if a person uses multiple strains during the course of the day, that person will spread out the TCP and, in doing so, expose the body to a more comprehensive treatment. This variability increases exponentially when adding different strains and using them in tincture, vaporized, and raw, and preheated cannabis capsules. Other forms add to this variability, presenting unique treatment features to the body throughout the day. Additionally, purposely using different strains in different forms, presented in different ways, maintains a paradox presented to the brain of simultaneous familiarity and novelty. This duality of opposites causes a pleasure response generated by hedonic hot spots in the brain. It also inhibits the body's ability to adapt around treatment.

The initial phase of treatment with medical cannabis is geared toward use of tincture to titrate up high-CBD doses during the day and higher-THC doses in the evening. Although many people develop symptom relief early on, the goal is to find out what is tolerable and to gauge initial symptom relief. In this phase, different embodiments are tried as time goes on, including vaporized cannabis concentrates or vaporized plant-based cannabis. The patient gathers information about what helps and what causes cognitive changes. They can then decide what they want to use and when they want to use it.

Focus shifts in the intermediate phase of treatment with the introduction of raw and preheated cannabis in capsules and increased numbers of strains used. The TCP really spreads out. In this phase, the patient should expect profound relief of their symptoms.

In the advanced phase, not only are we rotating the strains used, the embodiments they come in, and the mingling of local and systemic delivery, but we are adding other potentially helpful supplements, such as turmeric, cayenne pepper, raw cacao, and GABA. We are trying to maintain profound symptom relief by preventing the body from adapting around it, while working toward resolution of the underlying condition that caused the symptoms to occur.

Responsible use also requires that patients who pursue this course of care spend some time learning the provisions of their state's law. Congress remains in support of states determining their own marijuana laws. To stay legal, any individual must follow those state laws, or they will not be protected in their state or federal justice system. It is therefore strongly recommended that any medical cannabis patients, caretakers, and providers read and understand their state's laws. Some states require their medical cannabis patients to register with the state, but others do not. In states that do not require patients to register with the state, patients need to decide if they wish to do this or not. All states require physician certification for the treatment.

Collaborative treatment is an interesting idea that is evolving in traditional medical care, but is an essential aspect of medical cannabis treatment. Usually, physicians do not come to this treatment with any greater understanding of it than their patients. Many have less. Patients using this type of care have often gone to great lengths to conceal if from their doctors for fear that the doctor will disapprove or, worse, discharge them from their practice. Patients may understand aspects of this care, but get much of their advice from the least qualified people, who are only passing on what has been helpful for themselves or people they may know who use medical cannabis. In the next decade, the endocannabinoid system will become a featured aspect of medical training. It is a system involved in managing most chronic and many acute medical conditions. As greater medical knowledge leads to greater participation by physicians in medical cannabis treatment, patients will gain the general and personal health advice of their practitioners. Collaborative care involves both providers and patients sharing success and failure in treatment that is forged with both parties contributing suggestions and ideas.

Additionally, patients should be encouraged to try things beyond the physician's recommendations, because this is an extremely important component of figuring out what aspects of medical cannabis treatment will work for any individual.

Data collection and advancement of science are other hugely important aspects of medical cannabis treatment. Medical cannabis treatment has involved a lot of dedicated people helping each other out to determine best treatment. Similarly, people using Medical Cannabis should gather and share their own treatment outcomes with others and smartphone apps need to be developed to collect and analyze it. Dispensaries need to promote this data collection and should become places where studies are set up and run. Additionally, physicians need to encourage their patients to participate in the data collection. The only way for the science to fully advance as the treatment unfolds is with the collection of data and comparison of large data sets.

One of the challenges of medical cannabis as a treatment is to make it work with traditional medical care and complementary and alternative care. To do this, patients and their practitioners must come together to work on this treatment approach. Although physicians are required to certify people for medical cannabis treatment, anyone can make suggestions and ideas. For health professionals of any sort to do so, they must study the science and understand how the endocannabinoid and phytocannabinoid systems work together. Additionally, professionals should be aware of the various ways this treatment can be done, and the pros and cons of each approach. Patients have done and can do this treatment on their own, but collaboration can be a more effective approach. The rule with treatment is that there are no clear rules. Everyone responds differently and needs to determine what is tolerable and what works. Guidelines for treatment help to establish effective care, but ultimately it is the way that people innovate with this treatment that makes it most useful.

Caregivers and family members need to understand that medical cannabis is nothing like recreational cannabis. While the medical cannabis patient can be altered, it is not necessary to be altered any of the time for this treatment to work. Imagine telling someone who was using cannabis recreationally that the goal is to use it without getting stoned. And yet that is exactly what we can teach medical cannabis patients to do. No medical treatment can be truly successful if it makes the consumer altered all the time. Medical cannabis care is no exception.

This does not mean that either being high or use of THC, the main psychoactive phytocannabinoid, is undesirable or a side effect of treatment. It means that for treatment to work, a person needs not be altered by it when performing tasks or interacting with others. In states that allow caregivers to help with purchases at dispensaries, understanding the basic principles laid out in this book regarding proper treatment options is important. Hearing of people's personal experience with medical cannabis can be helpful, but is not specific to anyone else. Because the plants' properties and genetics are varied and human genetics have evolved with plant genetics, we are largely compatible with the plant, but everyone will respond uniquely based on the interplay of these genetics. One's personal experience with up to 111 phytocannabinoids in cannabis is very different than with stable, single-ingredient pills. While medical cannabis is more unpredictable and unstable than single-ingredient pills, it is also harder for the body to work around, in part due to the constant variation of what is presented to it. Different state laws have different legal restrictions for caregivers of people using medical cannabis. Many do not allow caregivers to purchase medical cannabis, but others do. This is another reason to review state laws if using this treatment.

The single biggest public health problem with medical cannabis is arrest, conviction, and incarceration of people who use this plant medically or recreationally. Marijuana's status as a Schedule 1 drug is absurd. It is a far safer recreational drug than caffeine, tobacco, or alcohol, and even counters some of the effects of those legal and lucrative drugs. That there is one person in prison or jail for simple possession is a true travesty of justice, and must be looked at through an ethical microscope and curtailed. To hear the private prison industry state that this must remain an offense punished by prison time to preserve its profits and viability is crass and repulsive. To sacrifice lives for this unfair and arbitrary criminalization of a plant that is this helpful medically, so that a questionable private prison industry should flourish, is the picture of injustice.

This picture is only amplified and distorted further when the demographics of who is imprisoned for marijuana possession is so skewed towards people of color. It makes a medical treatment for some a justification for race and class warfare for others. This is a social issue that so treads on the disenfranchised of all races that it must be ended. Medical cannabis as a treatment does need to be decriminalized but should not be scheduled at all. Doing so would put it into the hands of an ill-prepared community of physicians. It is a new treatment, and needs to evolve with greater physician participation, but should always remain patient-centric, not physician-centric.

It is also time for legislators to understand that this treatment is not about being "stoned" all the time. It is about developing more ways of using it without this effect. In the same vein, THC should not be eliminated from this type of care, because it is a highly effective medicinal phytocannabinoid that is needed both in its own right for many patients and to balance the treatment with non-psychoactive phytocannabinoids. Furthermore, the raw form of this plant contains little significant THC. Instead, it has the highly pharmacologically active THCA, which does not induce a high. It hampers efficacy of treatment to eliminate its contribution to providing a feeling of wellbeing while reducing symptoms of pain, spasm, inflammation, cancer, nausea, vomiting, and brain damage.

Some have argued that using a drug like cannabis to replace a drug like opioids makes no sense, but this completely misses the point of proportionality. Cannabis issues are not equivalent to opioid issues. To be sure, there are issues with medical cannabis, but no one dies from overdosing on medical cannabis. It does not cause brain damage in either adults or adolescents, according to the latest studies. While it can be highly abused (as can alcohol, tobacco, and opioids), many who use it recreationally do not do so. There are and will be others who do abuse it, but this is no reason to eliminate it as a medical treatment. Among the vast majority, there is no abuse, or abuse stops and is replaced with responsible use. To be clear, some will derail their lives through use, and it can certainly make emotional problems worse or better. This issue should be one for treatment, however. Criminalizing or severely restricting such a benign substance not only does not work, but it encourages the blight on our society of criminal underground commerce and its attendant horrors.

Another problem that legislators need to address is that of either state lawmakers or state medical boards making decisions about which conditions can and cannot be treated with medical cannabis. It is also important to address the restriction of this treatment to specific low THC levels. These are issues that need to be determined by a patient and their physician, based on science, not preconceived notions or overly restrictive laws. Legislators have a big responsibility to determine state law, based on fairness, constitutionality, and protection of the public. Looking at the facts with medical cannabis and not the precedence or fiction built around that precedence is of critical importance in determining new law.

Our legislators have an awesome and difficult decision to make, especially in situations that affect so many. This section is in no way a critique of these hardworking agents of social order and social change, but is instead a call to reasonableness and fact-finding in determining the future of this treatment. Listening only to medical board members who have not studied, researched, or treated with this method, and buying into the alternative truth that there is not enough evidence to support medical cannabis as a treatment is inadequate. The lack of clinical studies is a function both of the difficulty of doing these with such a widely varied plant and the active hindrance, at least until recent days, of authorizing these studies in a clinically useful manner.

At the federal level, the current "don't ask, don't tell" attitude will need to come to an end. The federal government needs to address the will of the people. With over 75% of the population expressing a favorable attitude toward medical cannabis, both houses of Congress will have to come up with some decision about drastically changing federal law and decriminalizing and legitimizing use of this treatment. This is one of the only issues with bipartisan support in the United States, and so the current prohibition of use of cannabis will inevitably end. Dealing with this thoughtfully and directly would be preferable, but the will of the people is legalization of medical cannabis. It isn't even close.

I am a physician, not a lawmaker, but I know that the main thing physicians and legislators have in common is their desire to help others. Over the next several years, physicians with knowledge of this subject and experience in treating patients must weigh in with legislators to make this potentially life-saving and life-enhancing treatment available to our patients. While individual states should continue to take the lead in passing laws to determine the details of this treatment, it is time for the federal government to look at the overwhelming efficacy and safety evidence, as well as the will of the vast majority of their constituents, to provide the overall framework of legalization of cannabis as a medical treatment.

There are many myths about medical cannabis treatment. These tend to be perpetuated from generation to generation. Many arise from the drive to grow and use higher-THC plant strains, but they have been applied to high-CBD plants, as well. The table below lists many of these and explains the best current understanding.

TABLE 18: MEDICAL CANNABIS MYTHS

Myth	Fact
To do this treatment a person will be cognitively impaired, altered and stoned	There are multiple ways to do this treatment with any strain of cannabis, without being impaired
This treatment is unhealthy because marijuana smoke has more tars than cigarettes	There is no evidence that smoking cannabis is a health risk and it does not need to be inhaled to be effective treatment
Smoking marijuana causes increased appetite and weight gain	High CBD cannabis is associated with transformation of white fat to brown fat and promotes weight loss
Specific strains of medical cannabis treat specific medical conditions	There is no evidence that specific strains work for specific conditions, but specific cannabinoids work for specific underlying problems like inflammation or pain
Cannabis Sativa strains give energy and Cannabis Indica Strains are relaxing	There is no evidence of this and these distinctions are actually just about THC dominant plants. Most cannabis species today are hybrids of Sativa and Indica
Marijuana can cause brain damage	Cannabis is neuroprotective and this is true for THC, CBDA and CBD
CBD is the good phytocannabinoid and THC is bad	Of the 10 phytocannabinoids with identified therapeutic action, the ensemble effect of them working together gives the best medical result
When harvesting cannabis, hanging plants upside down causes cannabinoids to drain to the flowers	Once harvested, cannabinoid production, location and transport are done and fixed. No cannabinoids will drain to the flowers

Myth	Fact
Raw cannabis is inactive and preheating, vaporizing or smoking it activates the plant	The raw plant offers acidic forms of several cannabinoids, many of which are actively medical
Tincture absorbs best under the tongue	At leas for CBD, under-the-tongue absorption is the least efficient

Medical cannabis is a treatment that changes over the course of a patient's life, moving through phases of care. Rather than look at what strain of cannabis is good for which disease, it is much more informative to review the properties of the phytocannabinoids (**Table 1**), and spread out and rotate the number of strains that can be used in the course of a regular day, without causing any alterations or impairments. This is further enhanced by using different embodiments of the treatment and different routes of administration. In the evening, higher-THC strains can be used to enjoy the psychotropic effects or mask them later in the night with sleep. In fact, using them for sleep is an appropriate strategy, as deep stages of sleep help power-wash the brain of the residue left behind from burning so much of the body's available energy. The three-pound brain uses 20%f of the body's daily energy intake. Stress reduction, improved quality of life, improved mood, improved pain, improved energy, and improved focus are all reasonable goals of this type of treatment. The treatment is compatible with the built-in endocannabinoid system, and this contributes to making medical cannabis treatment excellent at restoring health, wellness, and the pleasure of a life well-lived.